EasyFit: A Simple Guide on How to Look Better and Feel Great

AuthorHouse™
1663 Liberty Drive
Bloomington, IN 47403
www.authorhouse.com
Phone: 1-800-839-8640

I0412725

First published by AuthorHouse 9/23/2011

ISBN: 978-1-4634-6813-2 (e)
ISBN: 978-1-4634-4725-0 (sc)

Library of Congress Control Number: 2011914329

Printed in the United States of America

This book is printed on acid-free paper.

Because of the dynamic nature of the Internet, any web addresses or links contained in this book may have changed since publication and may no longer be valid. The views expressed in this work are solely those of the author and do not necessarily reflect the views of the publisher, and the publisher hereby disclaims any responsibility for them.

LIMIT OF LIABILITY/DISCLAIMER OF WARRANTY:
The EasyFit program is meant for healthy adults. Please consult your doctor before starting this or any other program of fitness and nutrition. The authors, producers, publishers and/or assignees take no responsibility for the results or lack thereof by participants, nor do they take responsibility for any injuries incurred to participants while following this guide and the programs it contains.

I would like to thank and dedicate this book to

Iris Wakefield

for the idea of creating EasyFit

and inspiring its completion.

credits and acknowledgements

PRODUCER AND COLLABORATING AUTHOR
David Wakefield

INSPIRATION
Iris Wakefield

AUTHOR
Sandra Dansereau

CO-AUTHOR
Jennifer Hruby

TECHNICAL EDITOR AND WRITER
Pauline Sebestyen

PHOTOGRAPHY
Blushing Peach Photography

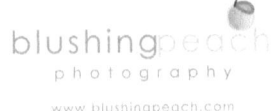

EXERCISES DEMONSTRATED BY:
Sandra Dansereau, BSc. KIN, CSEP-CPT
Kinesiologist

Jennifer Begg, CSEP-CPT
Kinesiologist

DESIGN BY:
The Print Shoppe

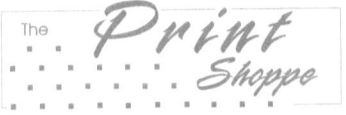

WHY EASY FIT?

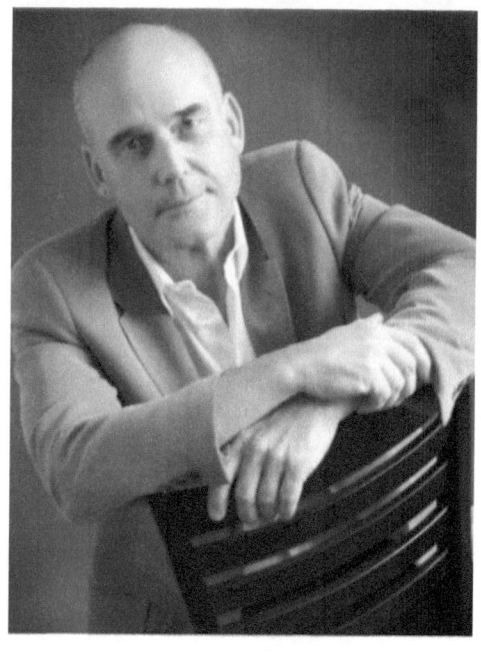

After 50+ years in the fitness industry, I wanted to provide an Easy way to help people look and feel better, no matter what a person's fitness level is. Whether you have ever exercised before or are in the shape you want to be, this program will work for you. By combining different exercises in the program, doing less or more based on your energy each workout. The idea is to get moving each week.

My goal is to offer a program that is available to use anywhere, in the home or while traveling, that can be easily followed with no equipment, no gym, and no hard-to-follow routines is identified in this simple guide.

The purpose of this book is to help enhance peoples lives and well-being through Exercise and Beneficial Nutrition.

In order for this guide to be most effective, I recruited professionals in both the fitness and nutrition industry to contribute their knowledge and experience in an area that is so often misunderstood or misguided.

SANDRA DANSEREAU, who has her Bachelors of Science Degree from the University of Calgary in Kinesiology and who specializes in fitness and wellbeing, is the author of this book. Her contributions to this book are well founded and proven to be very successful.

JENNIFER HRUBY, who has her Holistic Nutritionist R.H.N. from the Canadian School of Natural Nutrition, is the co-author of this book. Her valuable input provides knowledge on a healthy lifestyle through a well-balanced, nutritional regimen.

Both of these professionals offer the latest and most effective approach for getting great results using simple methods without expensive and unnecessary costs.

With EasyFit as your guide to fitness and nutrition, we are confident that you will benefit from this book and it proves to be an important part of your daily life.

As with all exercise programs a persons results will vary based on 1. the frequency - the number of times exercising per week 2. the duration of the program and 3. the intensity of the exercises performed.

I recommend three times per week - Monday, Wednesday & Friday or Tuesday, Thursday & Saturday - this gives a person 48 hours to recover from the session. This will vary based on an individuals schedule - you may want to mark the days down on a calendar - putting the time down also helps stick to the routine.

The duration of the program will increase as your fitness improves i.e. you may do number 1 stars for a while and then add 2 stars to the 1 stars increasing the time you are exercising. The stars are progressions that will be explained as you read on.

The intensity can be enhanced by doing the movements slower - 3 seconds 1/2 way through and 3 seconds completing the movement.

Bear in mind you always want to start off slow and progress as your fitness improves

David Wakefield

CONTENTS

INTRODUCTION

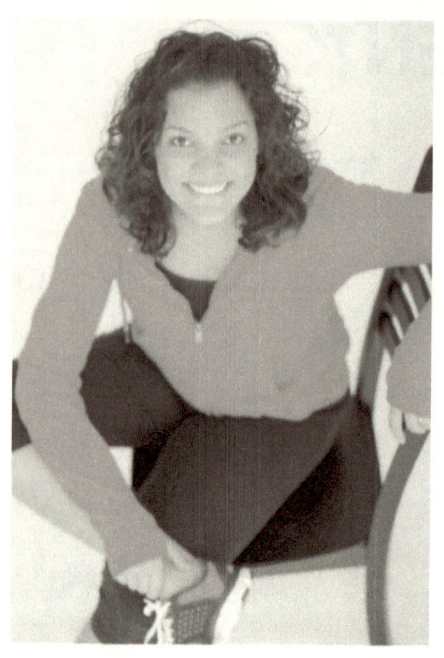

One of the biggest frustrations relating to the fitness industry is that programs are typically tailored for individuals who have a lot of time, money, and knowledge. Marketing ads, articles, commercials, and other sources of advertising focus on one thing—lose lots of weight and lose it fast! Even broadcasting companies are making money in this industry by means of reality TV shows that demonstrate drastic change in just a few weeks. But do these marketing methods hold true to their word? In reality, the average person does not have the time or money to drastically change their outer being using those same methods.

As an individual who has personally experienced the weight loss challenge, I have to say, "I understand what you are going through." I have battled weight since I was seven years old. At twelve years of age, standing only five feet tall, I weighed 180 pounds. There was a time when I would consume an entire bag of cookies and still head to the fridge for something more. My battle with a healthy lifestyle was both physical and emotional. So, when I say, "I understand," I'm actually holding true to my word. I understand through my own personal experience.

First, you cannot become a healthy person just by quickly losing weight. A healthy lifestyle does not come from a fast and "temporary" program. To lose weight properly, you must decide to change your lifestyle. This means a "permanent" change. I know that this may sound like a lot of effort, but the Easy Fit program is not like all the money-making gimmicks you hear about. Within this book, you will come to understand that fitness can be easy and fun, without burning a hole in your pocket.

Now, I am not going to lie and say that a lifestyle change is easy. What I can offer you is a good understanding—using simple methods—of how to improve your well being. It is important to know that improving your health is an on-going change, not a quick fix.

Working as a health practitioner, I have heard all the details and stories of why people are battling with chronic disease, obesity, depression, low self-esteem and all the other negative aspects that couple with low quality of life.

Another health issue I want to address is stress; specifically in the areas of occupation, spiritual, relationship, physical, mental and financial. Your emotional state ties directly into what you feel and how you live your life. If you feel stressed, you will most likely indulge in a favorite quick fix to feel better. Instead of fixing the problem by positively managing it, it is buried deep down and covered up with unhealthy habits. This is probably one of the biggest reasons why people indulge in food, alcohol or non-healthy addictive behaviors. If you are one of these people that practice this poor lifestyle, IT IS TIME TO CHANGE YOUR LIFE.

The tools and information that Jennifer and I have to offer will help you learn how to live a healthier lifestyle.

Sandra Dansereau

Easy FITNESS

Physical activity is movement. Movement is a behavior we lack in our society. Leading a life in a busy industry or engaging in a busy lifestyle can lead to unhealthy habits.

Not many of us engage in daily physical activity above and beyond regular everyday activities, such as gardening, walking or house work. It is great to continually engage in daily chores around the house, however, your body needs challenge and variety to keep healthy. This is because our body is a constantly changing organism.

When looking into physical and mental health, physical movement that increases calorie burn or heart rate can contribute to balancing the chemical processes we have in our bodies. When these chemical processes are overworked due to lack of exercise, issues can lead to chronic diseases such as obesity, diabetes, heart disease and so on. Much of the health industry focuses on body image and quick results; this can result in throwing our chemical composition out of alignment and make keeping weight off more difficult in the long run (such as yo-yo dieting).

When we focus on health, our aim is to concentrate on increasing quality of life and long term effects. So, challenge yourself physically and mentally everyday to contribute to a healthier lifestyle. Keep your muscles strong; ensuring, when you're older, you can walk without aid, stand up off the toilet without help, or recover easily from a fall. Keep your body balanced - by maintaining a healthy weight with appropriate fat levels— to contribute to a healthy environment for your internal structure.

This book will help support your first steps to a healthier lifestyle. You need to continually challenge your body, so remember this book is a stepping stone. When you get through and practice all of the eating and exercise routines, you should continue to challenge your body by using what you've learned and searching for other helpful sources.

When you begin to engage in a fitness routine, you should understand and consider your level of health. It is also important to keep track of your performance, since it helps to measure your progress of becoming a better you.

Fitness Benefits

Some of the benefits you can expect when engaging in physical activity are:

- Promotes the formation of muscle tissue
- Improves metabolism
- Improves circulation
- Decreases blood pressure
- Increases HDL (good) cholesterol
- Decreases LDL (bad) cholesterol
- Increases bone density, joint stability, endurance and strength
- Increases self esteem and self confidence
- Increases relaxation, mental alertness and sexual health
- Decreases chronic Injury
- Decreases pain
- Decreases developing disease
- Decreases stress
- Increases energy, decreases fatigue
- Decreases cravings
- Decreases excess weight
- Decreases/controls Type II diabetes

Importance of Technique

When sitting, standing or engaging in activity, the alignment of your spinal cord is important to maintain neutral. We have a natural curvature to our spine that keeps weight distribution equally on each vertebra.

Watch your body alignment, including:

- Ear
- Shoulder
- Hip
- Knee
- Ankle

Correct Posture

For the majority of day-to-day activity, our society is usually in a seated position; driving, working, watching TV or eating out are just some of many examples. As human beings, our bodies are not meant to be in prolonged seated positions. After a long time and as we age, our muscle imbalances worsen because we perform tasks in front of our bodies. Our heads slowly come forward (ear lining up with the front of our shoulders), shoulders curve in (sometimes resulting in our shoulder blades winging), and our upper back has a curvature development so significant that we begin to look like Mr. Burns from the Simpsons. As this continues down towards our feet, our natural alignment can begin causing pain in our lower backs, hips, knees and alter our gait (walking) patterns.

When engaging in any physical activity, it is necessary to maintain proper posture and exercise back muscles. This helps support weak muscles that have been weakened from sustained forward sitting posture.

While working out, maintain the key points during an exercise:

- Body alignment (ear over shoulder, over hip, over knee, over ankle)
- Double back to chest exercises
- Double tricep to bicep exercises
- Double quadricep to hamstring exercises
- Smooth coordinated and steady pace
- Abdominals contracted
- Engage gluts

These points are essential when working out, performing daily activities and strengthening appropriate muscles to support a better quality of life.

Bad Posture

Many people do not understand the long-term effects posture has in a healthy lifestyle. When our posture becomes altered—the chest is tight and back is weak—this can initiate many other issues physiologically.

Bad posture contributes to the following:

- Tight chest
- Shoulders pulled forward
- Collapsed rib cage, which means decreased amount of oxygen that goes into

the body since only 30% of lung capacity is being used

- Weak back, which promotes injuries and back ache
- No support for our spine
- Increase in pain because of prolonged unsupported positions

Importance of the Core
CORE MUSCLES (RECTUS ABDOMINAL, TRANSVERSE ABDOMINAL, LORDIS QUARDUM, OBLIQUES)

Why is it important?

The core abdominals seem to be the most neglected set of muscles in the body. More than 60% of Americans suffer from low back pain and sciatica. Fortunately, this can be prevented by appropriate posture and understanding on how to contact muscles to support the spine.

The gluteus and leg muscles are the biggest muscles throughout the entire body and, as a result, are contracted and depended on in order to carry out daily activities. The core is not necessarily just abdominal muscles. They are a combination of body muscles working together to ensure ideal supportive movements that the body can handle without causing a strain or sprain. In other words, these body muscles control smooth coordinated movement.

What you need to know about abdominals - for both men and women.

The transverse abdominals are the deepest set of abdominal muscles in the trunk. They represent a corset holding the spine in an appropriate strong, neutral position to carry out daily activities. This position holds your lower back muscles.

WOMEN

Women need to understand that core muscles not only involve the abdominals, legs and back, but also pelvic floor muscles. These muscles are also known as kegles; the primary muscle that women need to keep strong for labor and later on in life. Pre-mature urinary leakage and spotting, which occurs due to weak kegle muscles, is not normal. More women have this issue then you would think. These muscles become weak over years of not contracting efficiently during activity, not strengthening after labour, and from holding excretion outlets until you reach home (not using the bathroom when needed).

All these combined can cause increased stress on the pelvic floor weakening the muscles from holding your uterus in the upright position. The pelvic floor muscles also contribute to keeping the lower back strong (they connect to your lower back vertebrae).

MEN

The deep abdominal muscles are very similar to women but the pelvic floor muscles slightly differ. The contraction of the abdominal muscles and pelvic muscles still connect to the lumbar vertebrae. If these muscles are either tight or weak, they influence the health of the spine. If these muscles are tight, they will pull at the spine. If they are weak, they do not support a stationary position the lumbar spine requires to support lower back muscles and movements for lifting and carrying weighted objects.

How do you strengthen the core?

Strengthening these muscles is simple but tedious. At first, you need to perform this exercise throughout the day for two minutes and, at least, three times a day. It is important to maintain this exercise daily. You will progress to walking around holding this contraction and then while engaging in activities like lifting a weighted object, working out, running, carrying groceries, shifting a weight from a counter top to another counter and driving.

CONTRACTING THE TRANSVERSE ABDOMINAL:

1. The first engagement is lying on your back, with your knee bent and feet close to your bum, so that your middle finger can brush the back of your heel.

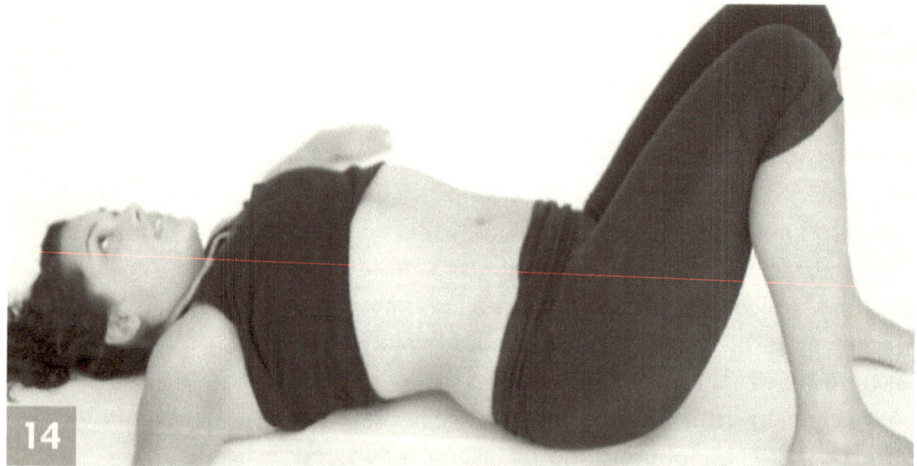

2. Try pushing your lower back into the floor.

3. Pull your belly button to your spine and breathe through the chest.

4. The tricky part is to maintain the stomach to be slightly drawn in and to breathe normally.
DO NOT HOLD YOUR BREATH!

5. Hold this exercise as long as you can.

6. You also need to contract your gluteus. This is the same feeling as holding in gas. Now contract those gluts until you feel the lower area engaging; SHAKING indicates you are doing it right. The first time you perform this exercise you may not feel anything, however, you will know that you are trying to engage something. These muscles are not use to the contraction and are working on the muscle neural system to respond to the demand sent from your brain. So don't worry, it will start feeling like you're doing something in the next couple times you do this exercise.

Starting this exercise is easier on the back then in any other position. Once this exercise becomes challenging and you are able to maintain a contraction over a minute, try the exercise holding up one leg. If your lower back rises off the floor, you are holding your leg too close to the floor. If this is the case, pull your leg higher up to support the position. After the exercise becomes easier, start to switch the legs while starting out with both knees up (straight above the hips). Then start in a squat position and then standing and then walking to running/jogging.

How do I know if my core muscles are weak?

You will know these muscles are weak if you cannot sustain the above mentioned exercise for at least 20 seconds without fatigue.

Additionally, women can check the strength of their pelvic floor muscles by positioning the pointer and middle finger together, inserting them in the first inch of the vagina opening, and squeezing the pelvic floor muscle. If you feel a slight squeeze, you have some work to do. A strong hold means you are strong, but need to keep up the exercises to maintain that strength. It may be a little uncomfortable to test this out, but it saves the possibility of many embarrassing moments or surgery in the future.

The Workout

Let's face the facts, we age every day. Our body goes through processes of oxidation, which basically breaks down our soft tissue to be replaced by brand new cells. If we do not exercise, our body becomes weaker than they were before and, since it adapts to lifestyle, it needs change and challenge everyday to increase strength, health, and endurance.

Working out is not everyone's favorite task, however, it does not require you to constantly "hit the gym". Working out is engaging the body in movements through all planes of motion such as dancing, walking, hiking, and simple practices around the house. The body is not supposed to maintain a standing and sitting posture. Our society supports our bodies to maintain these positions to survive. Supporting our bodies in a forward-flexed position increases the chance of injury and chronic weakening of our supportive structures (skeleton and muscles).

Do you ever wonder why there are so many people suffering from lower back pain, neck irritation and knee problems?

It is most likely because they are physically not strong enough to support their structure and body weight throughout the day.

Exercises

Exercises in this book are designed to create a full body exercise program. Depending on how much time you are willing to dedicate to physical activity on a daily or weekly basis, you can pick any of the programs mentioned below. These programs include upper and lower body programs for five days a week (full body) or three days a week (full body). In addition to these programs, make sure you try to engage in some sort of activity every day, even if this means taking a walk, playing with your kids, or doing an outdoor activity you love to do.

Note: When you are doing any of the following exercises using the chair, make sure the chair is secure (I.e. use a flat, solid floor and a sturdy chair that has a great base of support). When you distribute your weight on the chair, make sure your balance is sturdy and your position on the chair is supported before you start the exercise.

The excercises are listed as one (★) star to five (★★★★★) stars. One star being the least challenging, to five stars being the most challenging

The choices offer a complete body workout. Additionally there are a variety of other exercises to choose from that are not star choices, including the partner exercises.

Starting with the one star exercise for the initial workout and then progressing to 2, 3, 4 and 5 star exercises.

Your fitness level will determine which level you will be using. Eventually you may be able to do all levels in one workout. Start the program at your comfort level. Then progress slowly.

Exercising daily is recommended for 20 to 30 minutes. You may consider doing cardiovascular training and stretching one day and alternate with strength training on the other days.

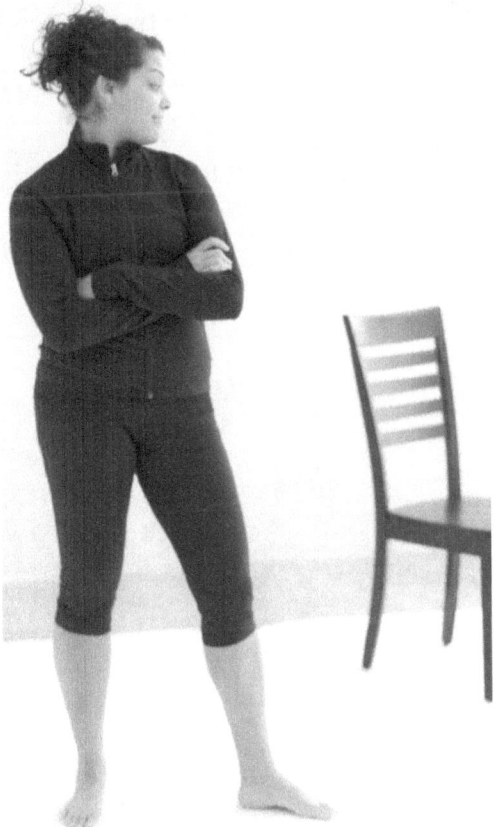

Your weekly exercise sessions should be part of your future weeks plans. Making an appointment with yourself at a specific time you have free.

A range of 8 to 12 repetitions per exercise is recommended. If you can do more than 12 then it is recommended you go to the next star level.

You can increase the tension by doing time under tension. Counting to 3 half way through the repetition and to 3 to complete the repetition (ie. 6 seconds per repetition x 10 repetitions = 60 seconds under tension.

Results will be achieved by the frequency, intensity and duration of your program.

CARDIO AND WARM-UP

Cardio or warm-up before any type of resistance training needs to be done in order to increase your circulatory system (blood flow), increase joint lubrication and elasticity of muscles. It is recommended that at least 15 minutes of warm-up is completed in order to effectively prepare the body.

The importance of warming up is to prevent injury.

★ Seated Heel Raises

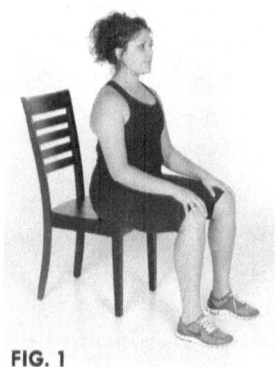

FIG. 1

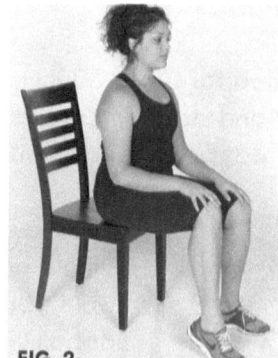

FIG. 2

Seated on the edge of the chair, place feet hip width apart. Start to shift weight onto left leg and lift the right heel off the ground, shift weight back onto the right leg and lift left heel. Continue until you feel warm. You can either place arms on your hips or leave loose by sides.

★★ Seated Side Slides

Seated on the edge of the chair, feet flat on the ground and sitting up tall; lift left foot onto toes and slide along floor. During this motion the body should remain still and slide foot as far to the side as possible. Return to start position and repeat on the opposite leg.

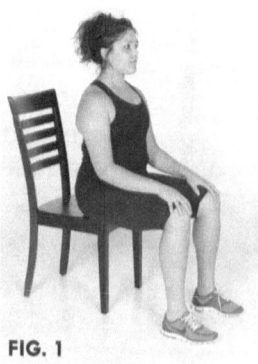

FIG. 1

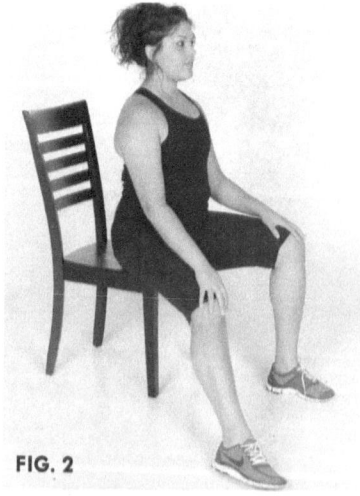

FIG. 2

★★★ Standing Side Steps

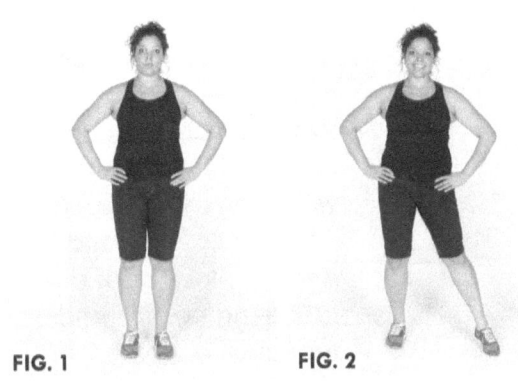

FIG. 1   FIG. 2

Standing tall and feet hip width apart; step left foot to the side, place back to start and repeat on right leg. Ideally continue until feeling of body temperature has raised or feeling of tiredness is present.

★★★★ Jumping Jacks

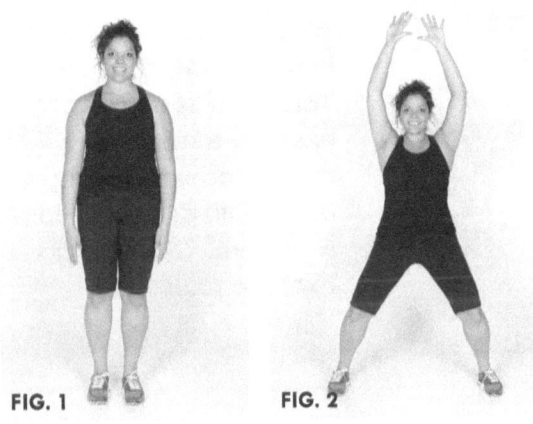

FIG. 1   FIG. 2

Standing tall, feet together and hands relaxed at sides. In one motion, jump feet apart and swing hands together overhead. Try to connect hands together and complete a clap.
Jump feet together and brings hands back to sides. Then repeat.

★★★★★ Flying Jacks

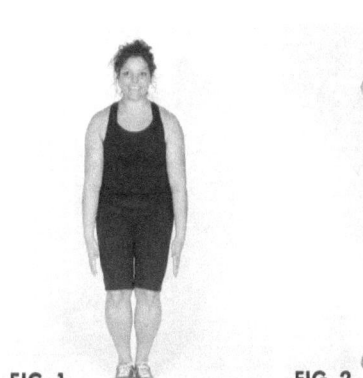
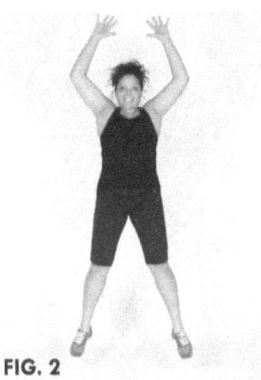

FIG. 1
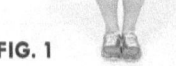
FIG. 2

Similar to Jumping Jacks; standing tall, with feet together and hands relaxed at the sides.
The difference is that you jump up from feet together and finish with feet together.

19

★ Seated Knees Up

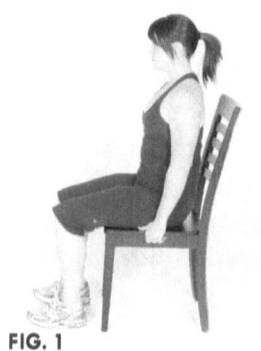

FIG. 1

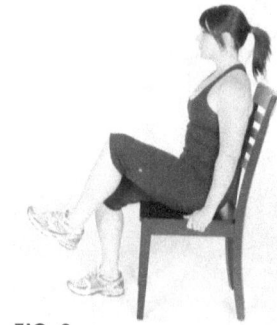

FIG. 2

Sitting on the edge of the chair, feet hip with apart and flat on the ground. Without leaning body back or shifting your weight onto one hip, lift left knee up (slow and steady), place back down to starting position and repeat on opposite leg.

★★ Standing Knees Up

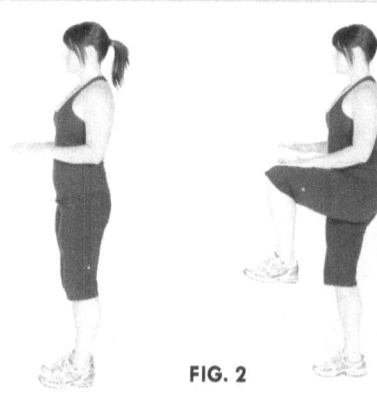

FIG. 1

FIG. 2

Similar to the seated knees up but completed in a standing position instead of seated. Each exercise should be completed until feeling of warmth or exhaustion is present. Ready to do exercise routine.

★★★ Marching

Standing in one spot, begin to walk, lift legs off ground and repeat one after another. Again until the feeling of muscles being warmed up or exhaustion.

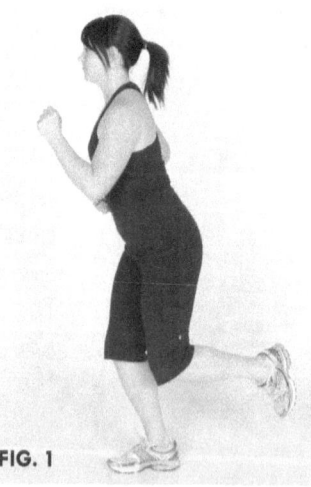

FIG. 1

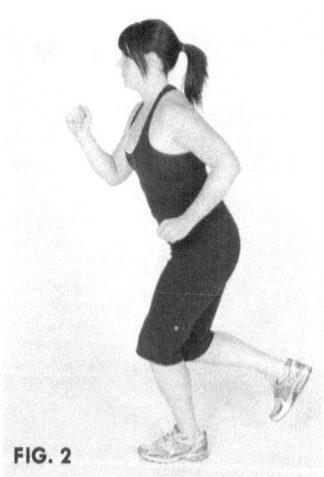

FIG. 2

★★★★ Step-Ups

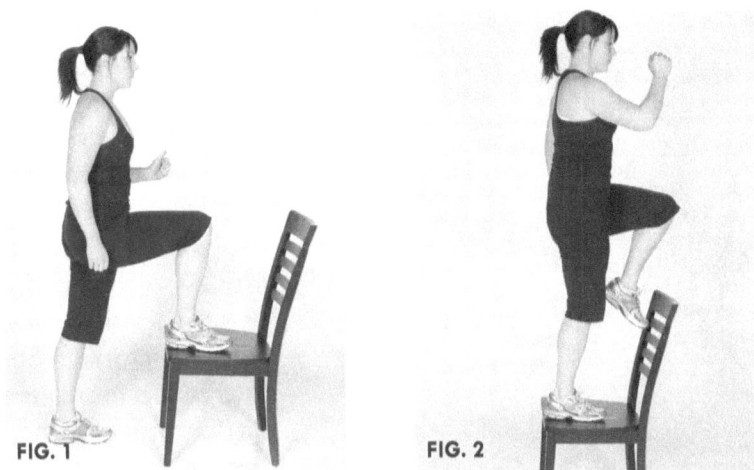

FIG. 1   FIG. 2

Stand facing a sturdy chair that will withstand body weight, place one foot on the chair. Engage core and gluts to sit body weight into the leg on the chair and slowly raise other leg off the ground to step onto the stair as well. Be careful not to bounce up to get the foot off the floor. Then slowly drop your foot back down to the ground while bending the other knee with control and technique.

★★★★★ Mountain Climbers

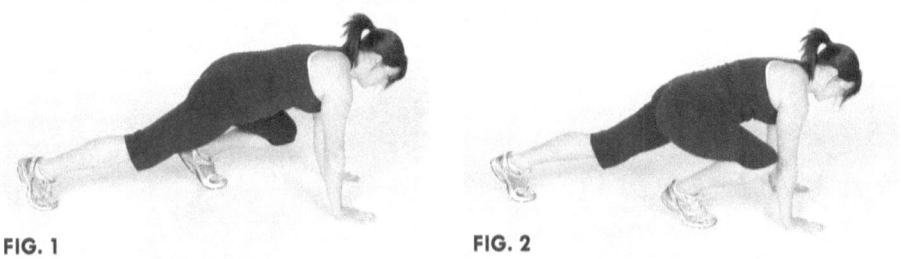

FIG. 1   FIG. 2

This exercise can be completed with hands on floor or on seat. The first step is to set body in a position that feels strong and stabilized; begin in a plank, pop hips up and jump one foot towards chest. Repeat by jumping foot back and bringing opposite foot to chest. Repeat until fatigued or maximum effort.

MUSCLES WORKED:
QUADRICEPS, HAMSTRINGS, CALVES,
ANTERIOR TIBALIS, GLUTEUS AND CORE

★   Forward Punch

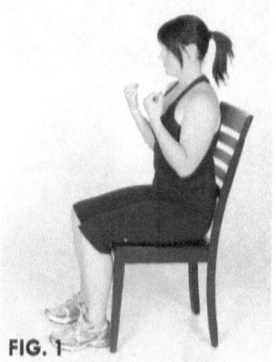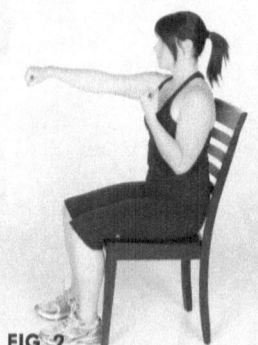

FIG. 1   FIG. 2

Can do this either seated or in a standing position. Feet flat on floor and fist at shoulder height, Elbows down at sides and standing tall. Punch forward with left hand, lift heel off ground as you reach forward and return to starting position and place foot back flat on ground. And then repeat.

★★   Punch Up (Seated or Standing)

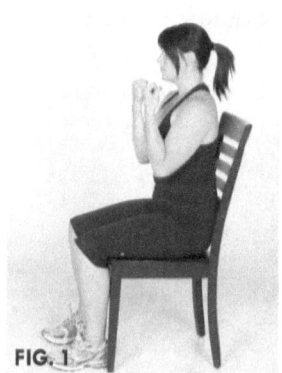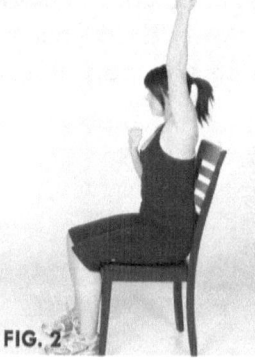

FIG. 1   FIG. 2

Similar to the forward punch, with fist at shoulder height and elbows relaxed to the sides. Punch up towards the ceiling, return to starting position and repeat.

★★★   Alternate Punching

Similar to forward punch, but alternate limbs and continue in a controlled faster pace. Make sure core is engaged and feet are moving with the punches.

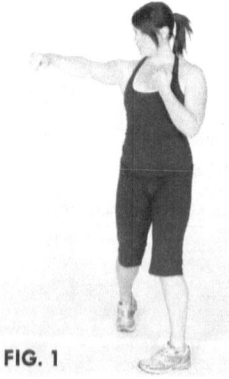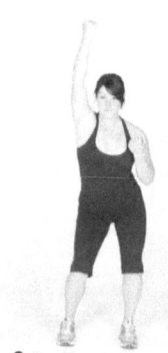

FIG. 1   FIG. 2

★★★★ Arm Pump

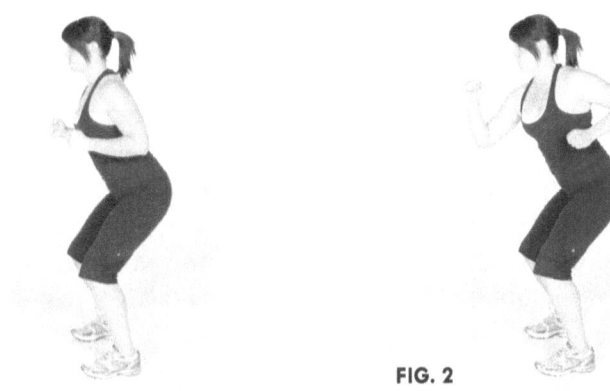

FIG. 1   FIG. 2

Similar to punch ups, but alternate limbs. Want a fast pace but control and keep core engaged, move hips and feet with each punch.

★★★★★ Speed Jabs

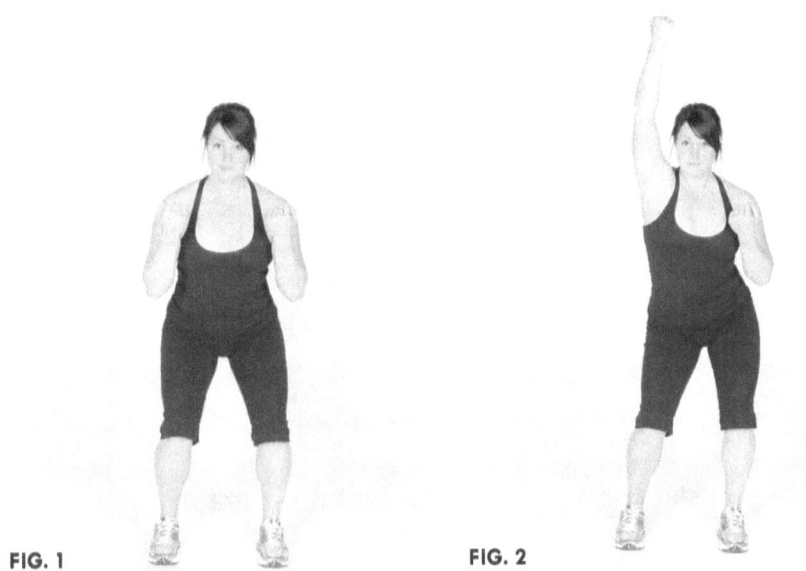

FIG. 1   FIG. 2

In the same starting position as the other exercises, drop elbow on left arm and punch towards opposite shoulder, keep elbow at 90 degrees and alternate arm. Repeat exercise.

MUSCLES WORKED: QUADRICEPS, HAMSTRINGS, CALVES, ANTERIOR TIBALIS, GLUTEUS AND CORE

RESISTANCE TRAINING
CHEST: FIVE STAGES OF PUSH-UPS

Even though our chest is tight from our everyday activities it is still important to strengthen these set of muscles. When doing the chest exercises it is very important to move in the full range of motion and move slowly throughout. During stretching it is very important to stretch longer on the chest muscles. Remember to keep your body balanced during your workouts, one chest exercise to two back exercises.

★ Standing Against the Wall

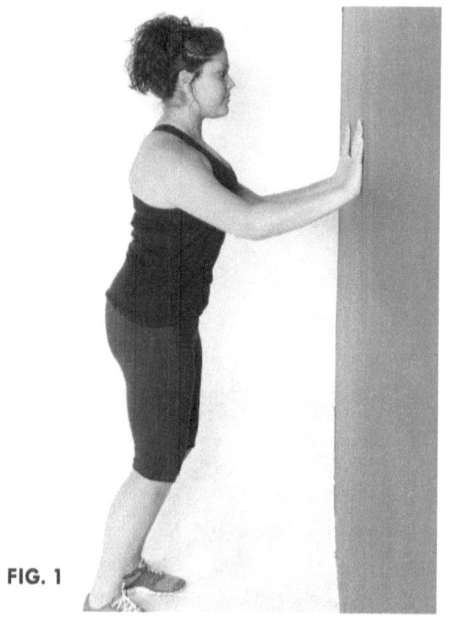

FIG. 1

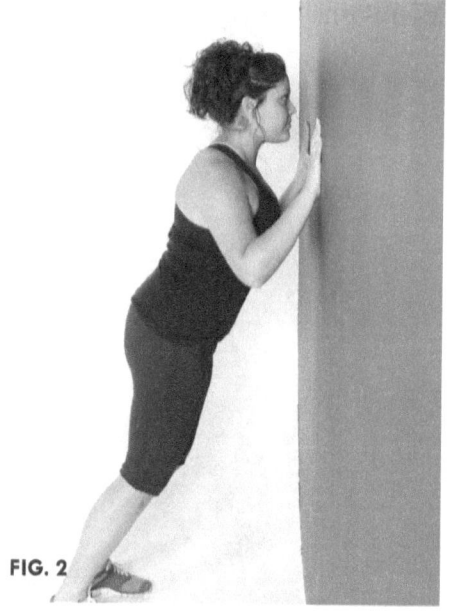

FIG. 2

Position yourself facing a wall and feet are arms length away. Place hands shoulder-width apart or just outside shoulder width. Shoulders relaxed and feet firmly planted on the wall. When ready, in a slow and controlled motion bend arms so elbows fall downwards towards armpits until you are close enough to the wall to steady your body weight and straighten your arms back to the beginning position. It is important to remember your boundaries to what you are capable of. You will know when you are ready for the next phase when you are able to touch your nose to the wall and slowly straighten your arms until you are in the beginning phase.

24

★★   Leaning on the Chair

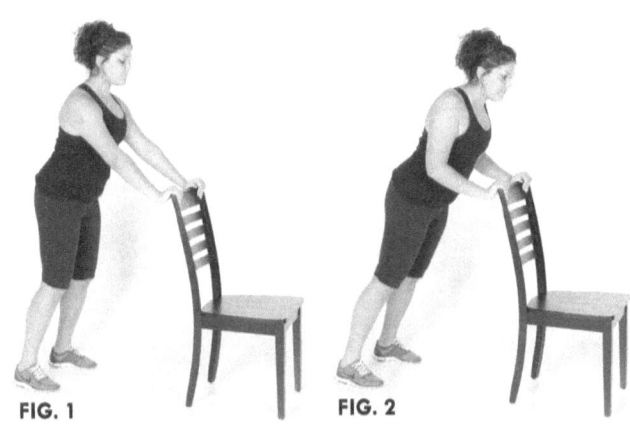

It is important to place the chair against a wall in order for the chair to stay in one place during this exercise. Place your hands on either side of the back of the chair and step back until you feel you are able to control your body weight. Slowly and steadily lower yourself to the top of the chair; elbows come towards the sides of your body. Lower yourself close enough to the chair to be able to steady and return to the beginning position.

FIG. 1   FIG. 2

★★★   Supine Straight Arm Flies

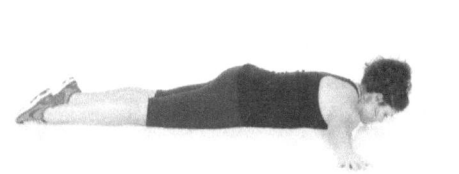
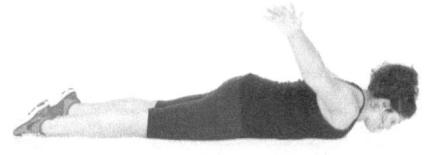

FIG. 1   FIG. 2

Start this exercise lying on your stomach or standing and facing the wall (your nose should almost touch the wall). Your whole entire body should be at rest with your arms straight along each side of you while you slowly with straight arms to each side of you. Lift your arms back as far up as possible until you feel your mid back contract. Hold this exercise for 3 to 5 seconds. Lower your arms in a controlled motion lower back to starting position and then repeat this exercise.

25

★★★★ Independent Towel Rows

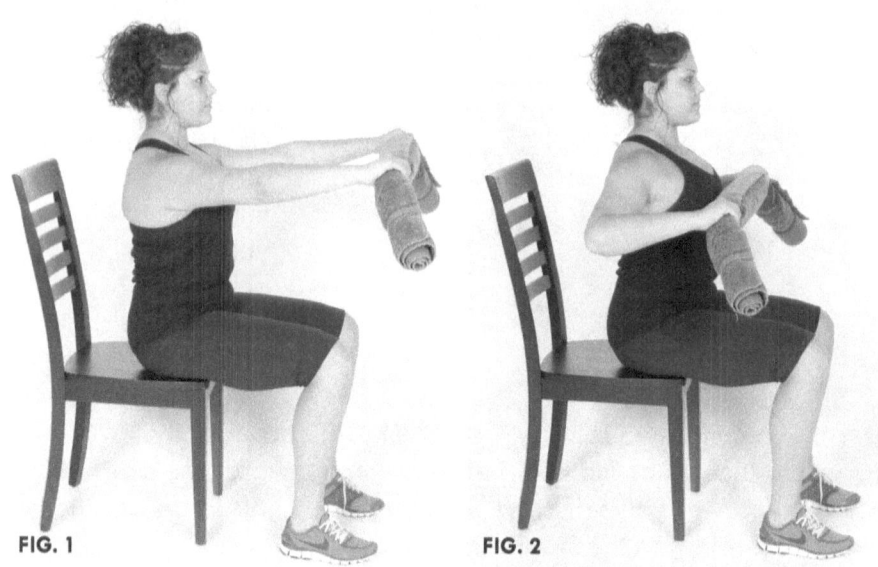

FIG. 1   FIG. 2

In the same seated or standing position as the first and second star exercise, hold a towel arms length away from you. Try pulling the towel apart and maintain this intensity. Pull the towel back towards you, elbows angling down along the side of your body with your shoulders relaxed. Squeeze your mid back and hold for 3 to 5 seconds. Then slowly return to the starting position.

★★★★★ Assisted Towel Rows

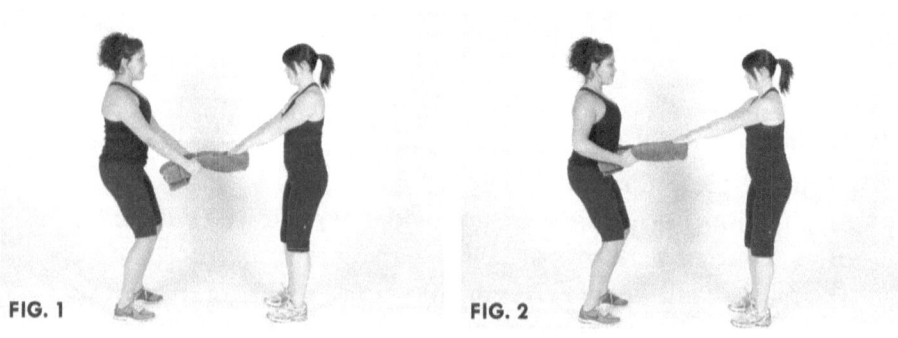

FIG. 1   FIG. 2

In the same motion as the fourth star exercise, have another person hold the end or middle of the towel to give resistance.

RESISTANCE TRAINING
BACK (MIDDLE/LOWER)

Similar to the upper/middle back strength any part of the back strength is ideal for optimal spine health, posture and injury prevention. The lower back is a connector between the upper back and lower extremities. The strength of this connection is important to recognize in order to understand that the back combination with the other muscle groups is how our body cooperates and moves together.

MUSCLES WORKED: LATS, SHOULDER AND CORE

★ Lat Holds

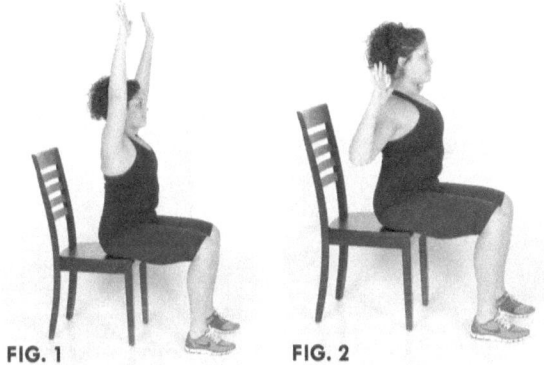

FIG. 1   FIG. 2

In a seated or standing position, hold your arms up as straight and comfortable as you can above your head. Roll your shoulders back, then bend your elbows and squeeze until you feel a contraction in the mid back. Hold this position for 3 to 5 seconds and then return to the starting position.

★★ Lat Pulls with Towel

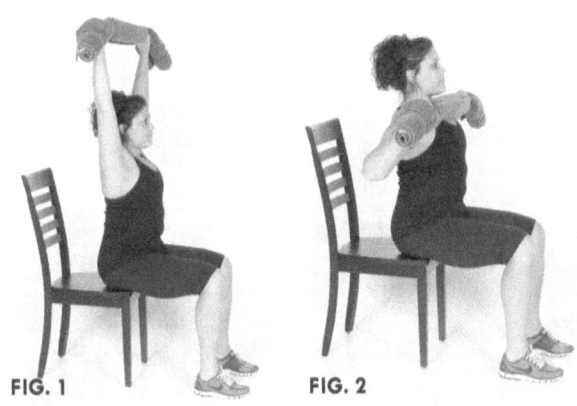

FIG. 1   FIG. 2

Follow the same instruction as the previous exercise, but perform it using a towel. Start the exercise by pulling the towel apart and repeat the same pattern of movement from the first star exercise.

Return to the starting position and repeat.

★★★ Inverted Push-Ups with Chair

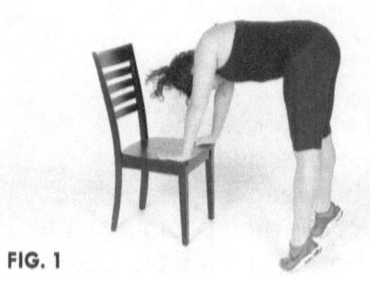
FIG. 1

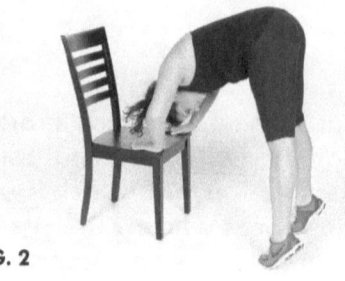
FIG. 2

Place your hands shoulder-width apart on the seat of the chair. Bend forward from your waist and move your body weight over your hands until comfortable. Bend elbows to slowly lower your head between your arms. Your goal is to get your head as close to the chair as possible with control. Straighten your arms and repeat.

★★★★ Inverted without Chair

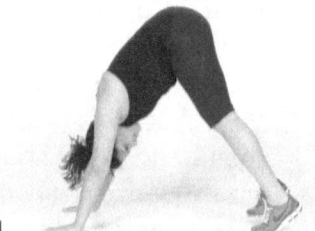
FIG. 1

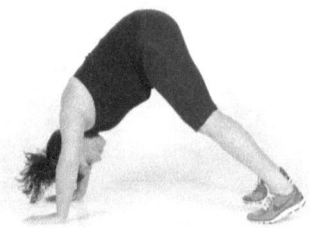
FIG. 2

This exercise is the same as the previous exercise but without using a chair. Stand up tall and bend over to place your hands on the floor. Your feet and hands should be far enough away to be comfortably placed on the floor without strain. Repeat this exercise and remember to control the movement.

★★★★★ Inverted Feet on Chair

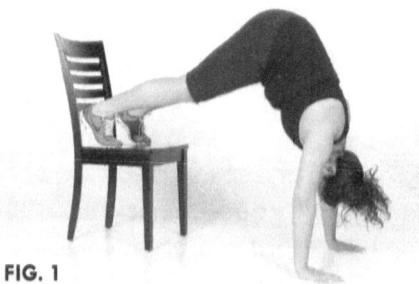
FIG. 1

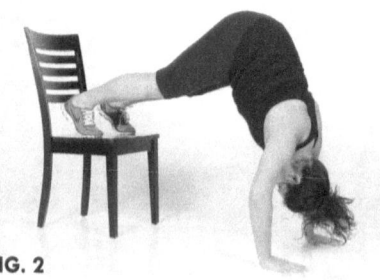
FIG. 2

Same as the previous exercise but place your hands are on the floor and your feet are on the chair.

RESISTANCE TRAINING
BUTT

Of course everyone loves a firm backside, but this is also important for smooth and coordinated movement. Did you know that your butt is the biggest muscle in your body? And not many people know to activate this during everyday activity. Your backend increase stability, strength and support for your spine. Standing up straight and keeping a strong mid-section is ideal for fantastic spine health, prevention of back injuries and supporting optimal posture.

MUSCLES WORKED: GLUTEUS MAXIMUM, HAMSTRINGS, TRANSVERSE ABDOMINALS, QUADRATUS LUMBORUM

★   Bum Squeezes

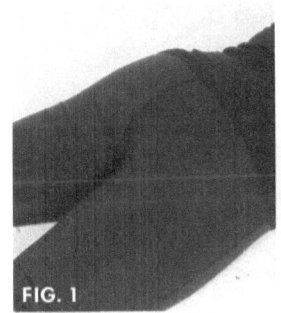

FIG. 1

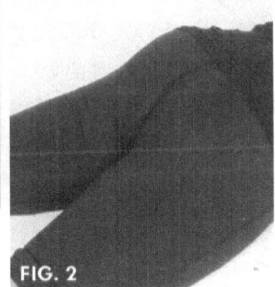

FIG. 2

Laying on your stomach (if comfortable) or in a seated position, clench your butt cheeks together, almost the same sensation as holding in a fart. Hold this exercise for 3 to 5 seconds and repeat.

★★   Standing Leg Extension with Bum Squeeze

Standing facing a wall, clench your butt until you cannot continue a contraction. Centre your weight so you are balancing on one leg. Keeping one leg straight, pull your leg away from the wall, hold for 3 to 5 seconds and return to the starting position.

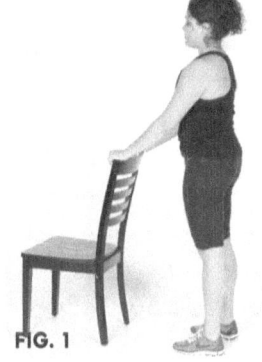

FIG. 1

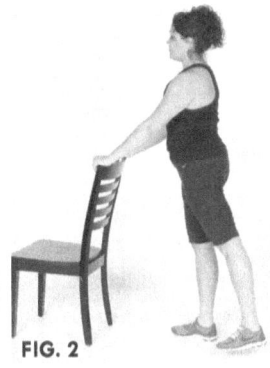

FIG. 2

★★★ Put Heels into Ground and Squeeze Butt

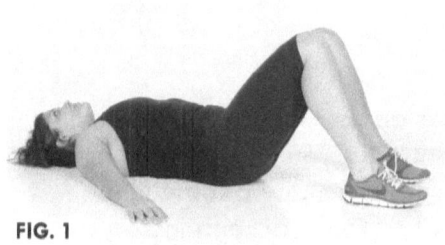

FIG. 1

Laying on your back, keep knees up and feet flat on the ground. Engage your core muscles, squeeze your bum (as if holding in a fart) and push heels into ground. Hold for 5-10 seconds, relax and repeat.

★★★★ Lift Bum

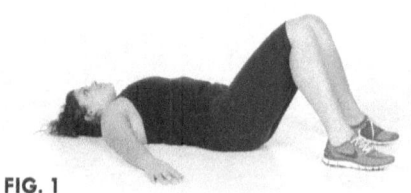

FIG. 1

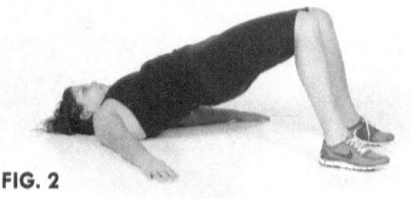

FIG. 2

Similar to the above star *** exercise but instead of engaging muscles and not completing exercise, lift bum up during the contraction of core muscles, bum and legs. With all exercises remember to control movement and move slow. Want to have a 1-2 pace during up and down phase of the exercise. Place your hands to your sides and palms flat on floor. Lift your hips off the ground. Your body should create a straight line from your knees and shoulders.

★★★★★ Back Bridge off Chair

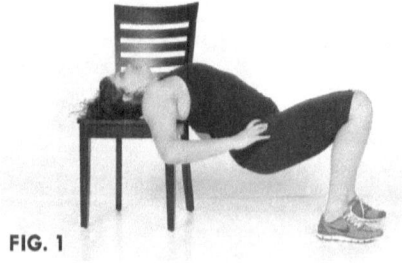

FIG. 1

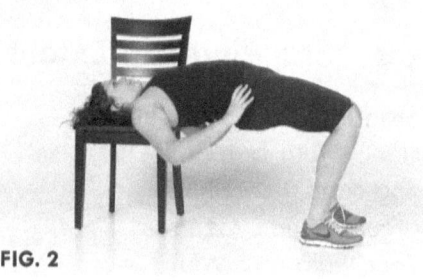

FIG. 2

This exercise can be with back on seat of chair or feet on seat of the chair. At first make sure the chair that would be used is sturdy and secure. Start with either your back or feet on the chair and opposite side of the body is secure on the floor. During the beginning of the exercise relax gluts and then engage. The ultimate goal is to keep body sturdy and contracted. Hold for 5-10 seconds, relax and repeat.

RESISTANCE TRAINING
CORE (ANTERIOR)

Anterior/front side of the body is very important to help support our core (ie. Our spine health). Isometric exercises are very important to combine with core exercises. It is important to remember to contract the three main muscle areas: Gluts, Transverse Abdominals and Pelvic wall muscles.

MUSCLES WORKED: TRANSVERSE ABDOMINALS, OBLIQUE, QUADRATUS LUMBORUM AND RECTUS ABDOMINAL

★ TA Contractions

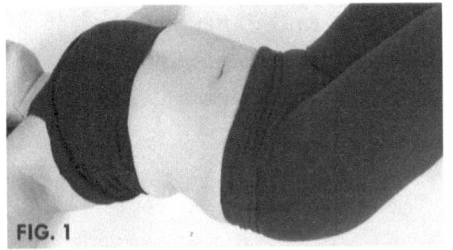 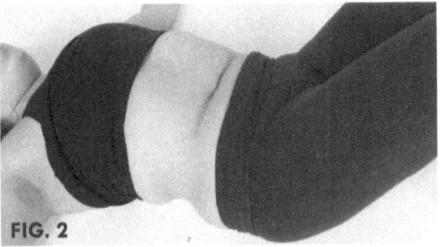

FIG. 1   FIG. 2

Lay on back with knees up and feet flat on floor. The key to transverse abdominals contraction is to keep everything contracted and held for 5-10 seconds. Keep entire back on floor (including lower back), pull belly button towards spine and contract gluts (similar sensation as holding in a fart).

★★ 4-Post Plank Until TA Engage

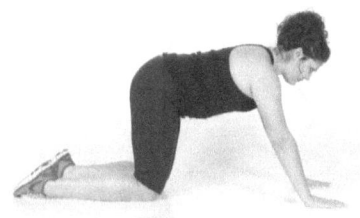 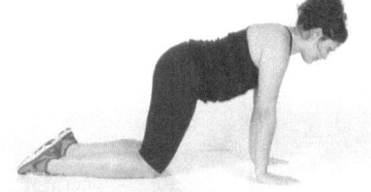

FIG. 1   FIG. 2

Start on hands and knees, keep hands and knees shoulder width apart. Stabilize all joints and hold transverse abdominal contraction for 5-10 seconds, relax and repeat.

★★★ Plank from Knees

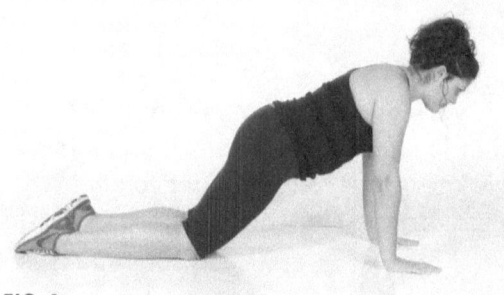

FIG. 1

The front plank is an isometric hold for the entire body. Begin by positioning your body on your hands and knees. Place your elbows just below your shoulders, while also bringing your body forward to bear weight through your elbows. TA contractions engaged and your trunk/thighs should hover above the floor. Your body should feel suspended between your hands and knees. Refer to the pictures to mirror the body position to yours. When you first try this position you may feel it is easy. If that is the case, well you're not doing it right! You should feel your trunk engage, pelvic tilt forward so you feel your abdominals engage and gluts activated. If you are positioned appropriately and don't feel it challenging, you then lift your knees off the ground and bear weight through your toes.

★★★★ Plank from Toes

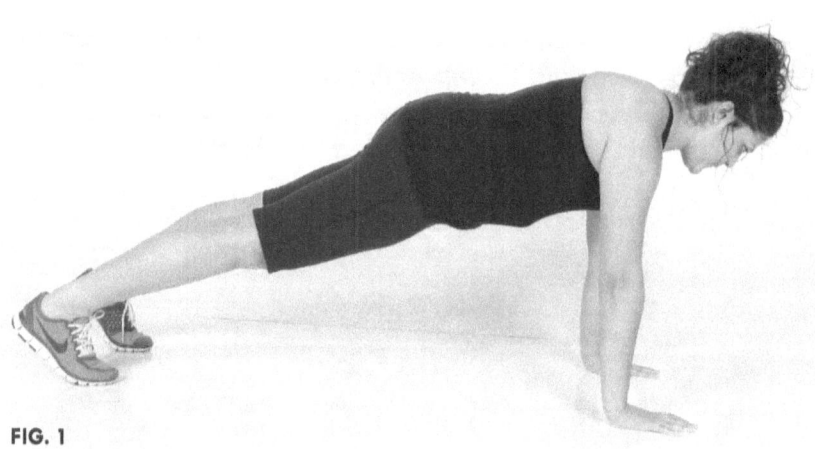

FIG. 1

Plank from your toes is similar to the plank from your knees. Keep transverse abdominals contracted throughout exercise. Only hold exercise for as long as the exercise is sustained without the presence of pain.

 ★★★★★ Plank with Toes on Chair

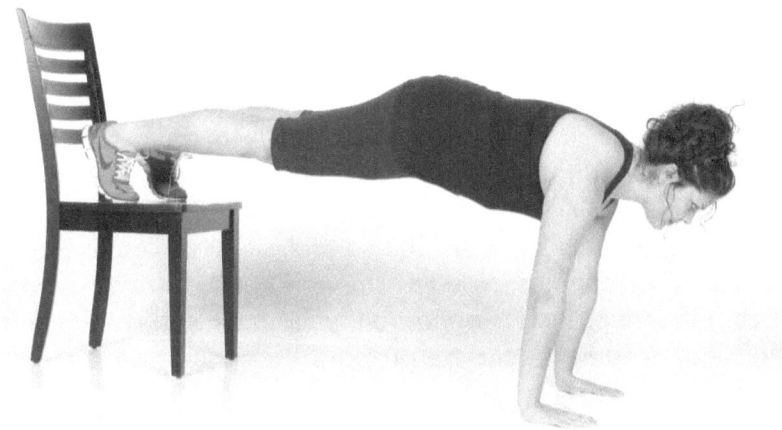

FIG. 1

Keep weight on hands; place one foot on the seat at a time, steady
body weight and engage core exercise.

Support your body weight by lying on your side. Place your elbow
directly under your shoulder and bring your feet towards your bum
(similar to curling up). Once you feel sturdy, lift your hips from the
ground and push hips forward to make a straight line from your
shoulder and knee. This is the first position, the easiest position. As
you feel stronger, balance off your feet instead of knees, then once
that feels stable then onto your hand and follow the pictures to the
hardest position. Planking from the chair will be easier then on the
floor. If you feel that it is hard to sustain a plank on the floor,
begin on the chair.

32

RESISTANCE TRAINING
CORE (POSTERIOR)

It is important to remember that when completing a back exercises that the TA and gluts are contracted throughout movements. Especially when arms are extended overhead, try to pull shoulders down and control movements. Also remember that speed is not efficient when doing exercises, slow and controlled is what we need in order to increase strength. The controlled movement is better in order to not only increase the strength but the stability of the muscles; this helps increase the ability for the muscles to adapt to unfamiliar movements and be prepared for unusual circumstances that can result in injury.

MUSCLES WORKED: BACK (UPPER AND LOWER), GLUTS, SHOULDERS AND LEGS

★ Against Wall Arm/Leg Extensions

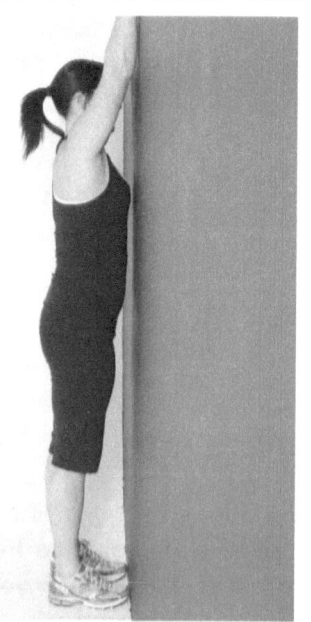
FIG. 1

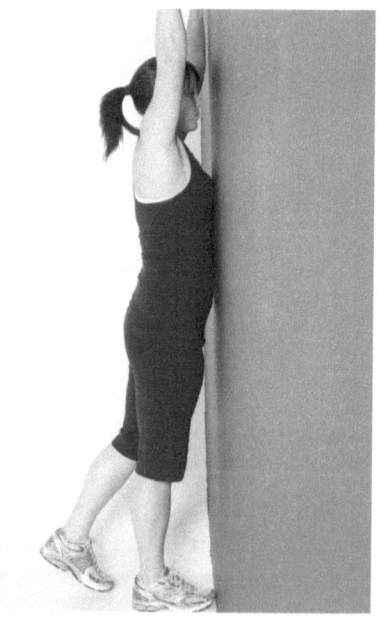
FIG. 2

Standing facing a wall, engage core, keep weight distributed evenly, and raise arms up above head. When ready contract opposite limbs and pull back, hold 5 seconds, relax and repeat on opposite side.

★★ Hands & Knees Supermans

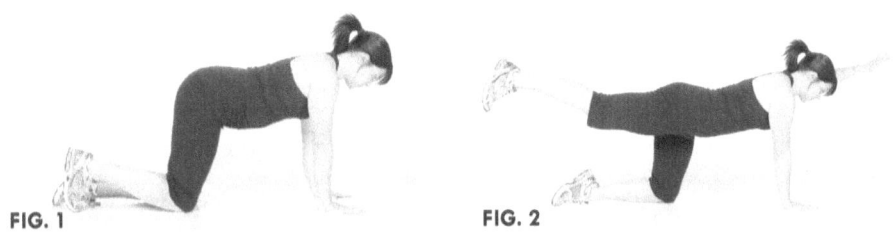

FIG. 1   FIG. 2

Begin on hands and knees. Engage TA, hands shoulder width apart, and knees hip width apart. Keep weight evenly distributed through trunk so weight will not shift side to side during exercise. When ready and core is engaged, lift opposite limbs toward the ceiling; keep thumb towards ceiling and foot flexed. Engage movement, hold 5 seconds, relax and repeat on other side.

★★★ Belly Supermans

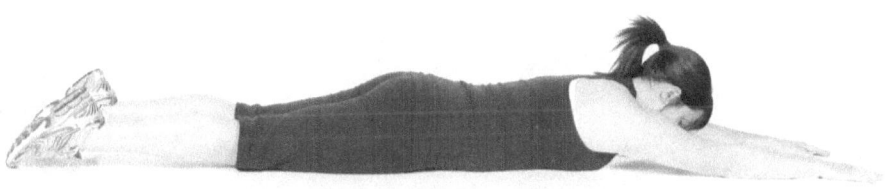

FIG. 1

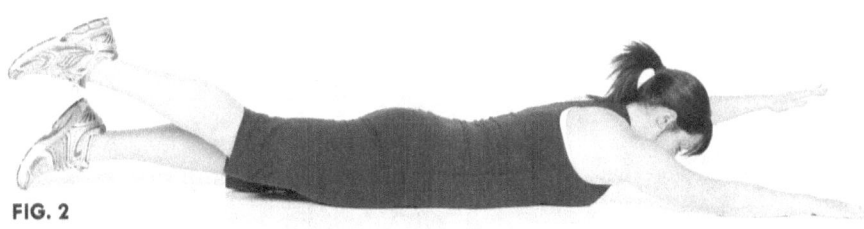

FIG. 2

Beginning on your stomach, relax your legs and your arms on the floor. Engage your core and back and lift your arms and legs off the ground towards the ceiling, hover and relax. This is a straight up-and-down movement, basic but effective.

MUSCLES WORKED: BACK AND GLUTS

FIG. 1   **FIG. 2**

Beginning on your stomach, relax your legs and arms on the floor.
Engage your core and back and lift your arms and legs off the
ground towards the ceiling, hover and relax.
This is a straight up-and-down movement, basic but effective.

MUSCLES WORKED: BACK AND GLUTS

★★★★★   Swimmers

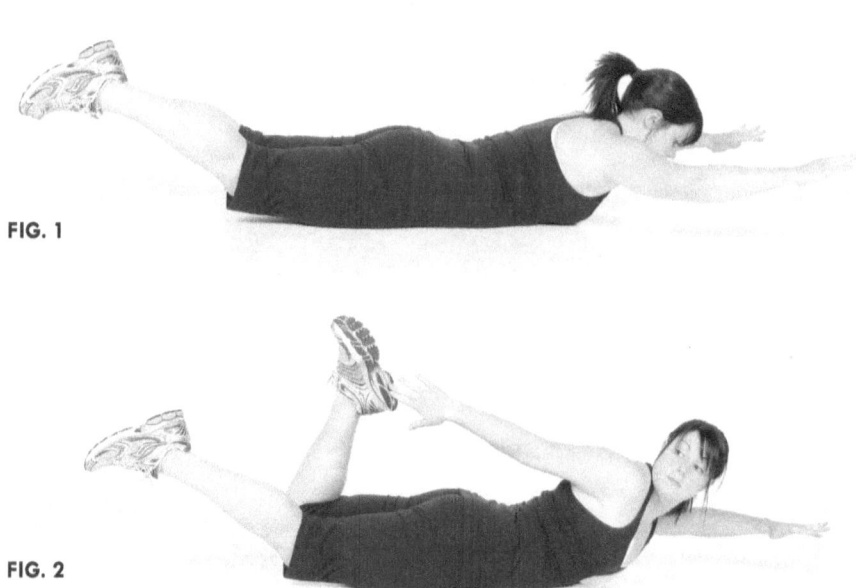

FIG. 1

FIG. 2

Similar to the cobra and starfish exercise, begin on your stomach.
Lift your arms and legs off the ground, bend elbows at 90 degrees
and level your shoulders. Bend your knees and keep your thighs
lifted off the floor. Engage your core and back. Look behind you
and try to aim one of your elbows towards the opposite foot. Slowly
return to start position and alternate to the other side.

**MUSCLES WORKED: BACK (UPPER AND LOWER),
GLUTS, SHOULDERS AND LEGS**

RESISTANCE TRAINING
QUADRICEPS (LUNGE)

Anytime a movement with the lower body is engaged, it is really important to engage all core muscles to keep support and increase stability to joints, such as the spine. Also remember when completing a lunge, the front leg is to stabilize movement and the back leg is to carry the weight throughout the exercise. Before proceeding into the exercise, make sure your body alignment is accurate. Are your hips square? Do your knees align with the outside of your hips? During the movement do your knees stay aligned or do they rotate towards the other leg? These are important tips while doing any exercise. Not following appropriate alignment during exercise can increase muscle imbalances already present from prior everyday cheating habits.

MUSCLES WORKED: QUADRICEPS, HAMSTRINGS, CALVES, GLUTS AND CORE

★   Supported Lunge by Hanging on to Chair

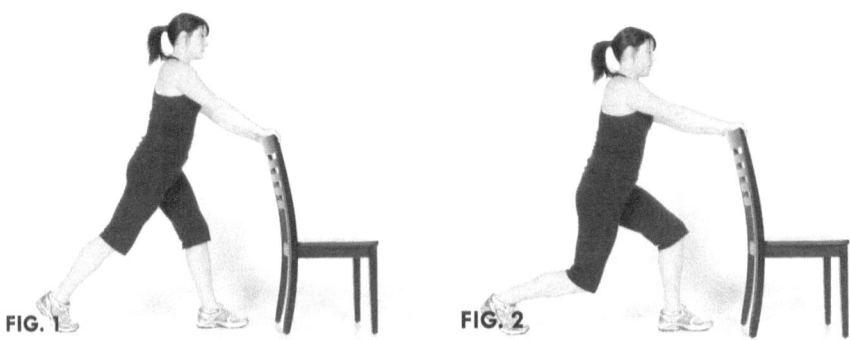

FIG. 1   FIG. 2

Standing beside a chair with your hand on the top of the back of the chair, step one foot as far forward as comfortable to begin exercise. Make sure weight is distributed throughout the back leg and the front leg is balancing the movement. Bend knees, keep knees 90 degrees, steady and return to standing, repeat.

★★　Balance Lunge

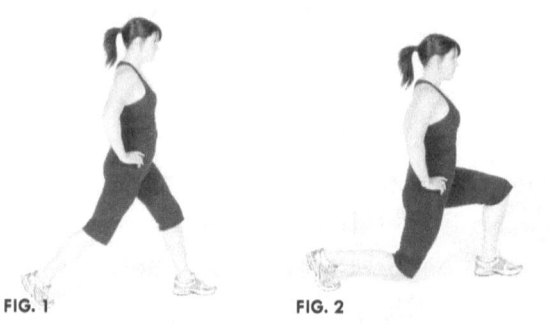

Stand with your feet separated, one behind and the other out in front. Your toes should be directed straight in front and your posture engaged. Bend both of your legs so the knee of the front foot does not pass your toes.

FIG. 1　　FIG. 2

★★★　Front Leg on Chair

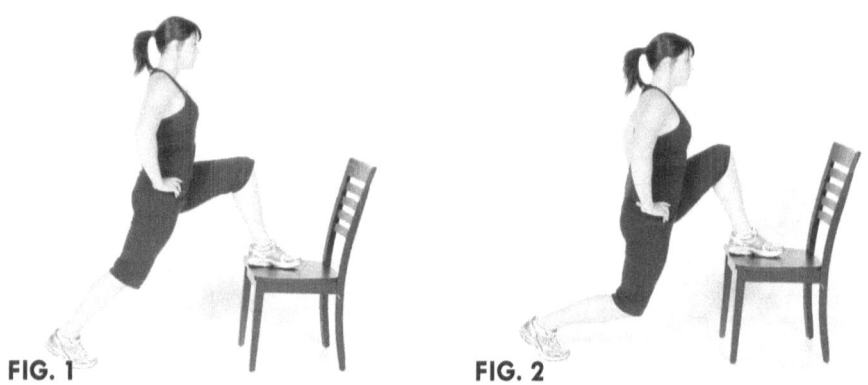

FIG. 1　　FIG. 2

Similar to lunges above, but front leg is positioned on chair. Make sure balance is secure before starting exercise. Lower body to the lowest position that is controlled and return to starting position, repeat. Then pick repetitions of 10x or 15x, and then switch legs.

★★★★ Back Leg on Chair

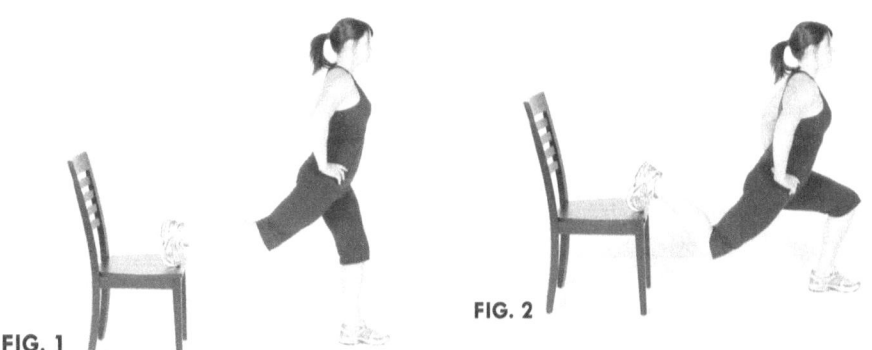

FIG. 1

FIG. 2

Similar to all lunges but back foot on the chair. Make sure balance is maintained throughout exercise. It is important to be able to keep movement slow and controlled to increase muscle recruitment and balance.

★★★★★ Split Jumps

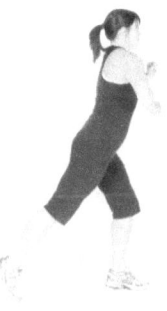

FIG. 1

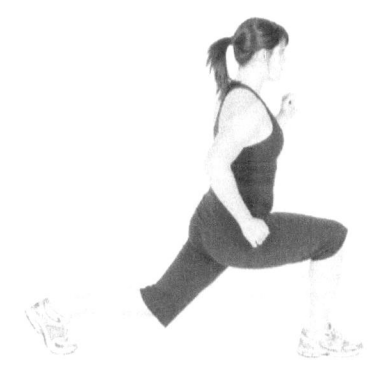

Standing up tall and arms relaxed to each side. Jump up and split legs, land in a

FIG. 2

lunge; jump up from the lunge position and switch legs. Use arms to help pump and increase momentum during exercise.

RESISTANCE TRAINING
HAMSTRINGS (SQUATS)

Unfortunately with our everyday habits, our hamstrings are usually the tightest muscle without maintenance exercises, such as everyday stretching. During many lower body exercises it is still important to increase strength and stability of any muscles, as in many are concerned with increasing their strength and think that this might increase the "tightness" but instead we need to focus on the full range of motion. When doing the exercise, we need to gradually go into the lowest squat possible without losing our balance. Gradually if this is possible being able to rise from a low squat, where literally your butt is a few inches off the ground and then into standing; this ideally is what everyone needs in order to maintain a high quality of life as we age. In our industry we understand that having a strong lower body and smooth functional movement is necessary for easy movement and recovery after a fall or broken hip.

MUSCLES WORKED: HAMSTRINGS, QUADRICEPS, CALVES, GLUTS AND CORE

★ Push Heels into Ground

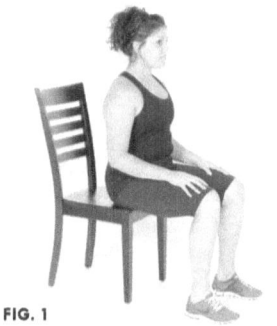

FIG. 1

Seated on the edge of the chair, sit tall, feet flat on ground and hands relaxed on legs. Engage core muscle, push heels into ground, hold 5-10 seconds, relax and repeat.

★★ Assisted Squat

Standing behind chair with hands on the back of the chair, place feet hip width apart, engage core muscles, keep weight throughout feet and bend your knees. During the movement keep knees aligned with ankles and push bum back. Keep chest up and look straight ahead during down and up phase of exercise.

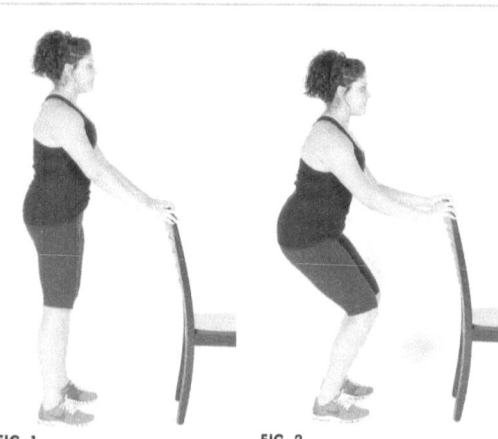

FIG. 1

FIG. 2

39

★★★ Get Up and Down Out of Chair

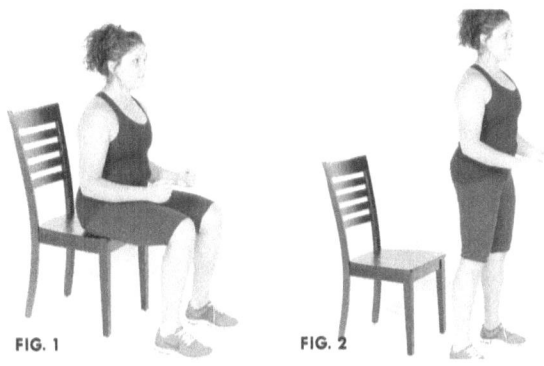

FIG. 1 FIG. 2

Stand facing away from the chair but only a foot away from it. Your feet should be shoulder-width apart and your arms relaxed to the sides. Slowly bend your knees as you would to sit into the chair. Slowly raise your arms up in order to balance body weight and create a smooth movement. Only lower body weight low enough for your thighs to be parallel to the floor. Then stand up. Repeat.

★★★★ Squat

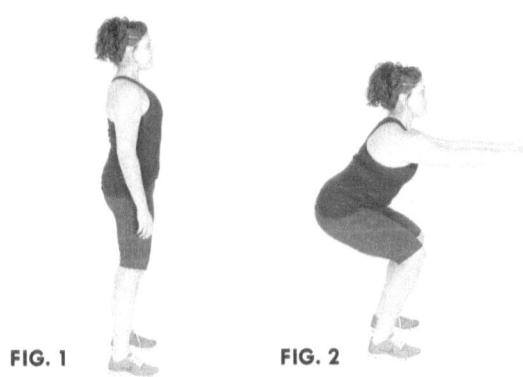

FIG. 1 FIG. 2

Similar to the exercise with the assisted squat. It is the same but no help with balancing during exercise. This exercise core is very important to maintain during movement because of no extra support such as a chair during movement.

★★★★★ Jump Squat

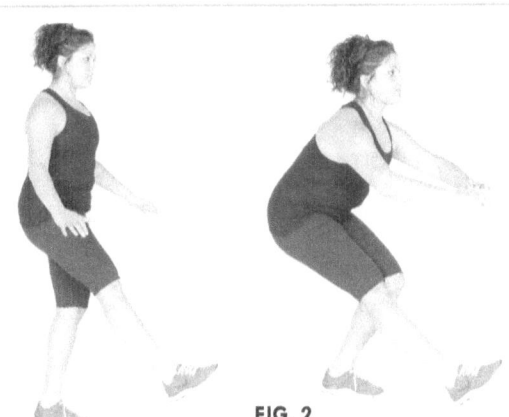

FIG. 1 FIG. 2

Same as squat but instead of just standing up into the starting position, jump up from the lowered position, land in the lowered bent knee position and repeat.

40

RESISTANCE TRAINING
BICEP

During any bicep exercise the posture in which you are standing or seated is important to maintain for efficient movement. When completing a bicep curl no movement in the body should be engaged; this is a form of cheating. When engaging in upper body movement it is important to not move the body, this will create other muscles other than the biceps to be engaged. Again it is important to move throughout the full Range of Motion, completely extend the arms and contract until your hand touches your shoulders.

★   Arm Pumps

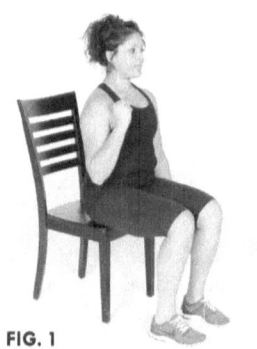

FIG. 1

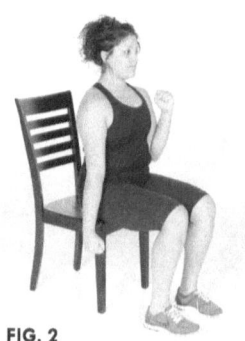

FIG. 2

In a seated or standing position engage core, make fists and keep them aligned at shoulder height and elbows relaxed at side. Straighten one arm while keeping the other positioned at shoulder height. Flex arm to return fist to shoulder height and alternate arms. Continue alternating arms with controlled and slow coordinated movement.

★★   Isometric Holds

In a seated or standing position, engage core, use the opposite arm in order to maintain contraction. The same movement as arm pumps, the opposite keeps the arm in motion from completing exercise, hold 5-10 seconds, relax and repeat.

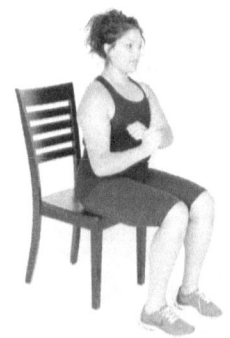

★★★ Eccentric Holds

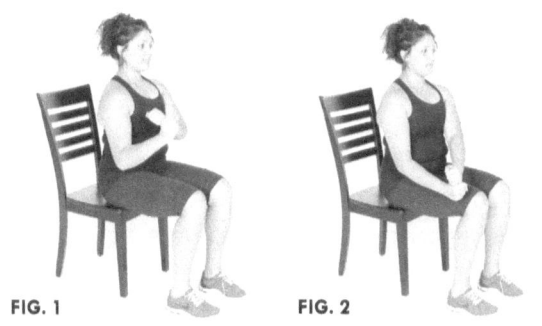

FIG. 1　　　FIG. 2

Same movement as the arm pumps and isometric holds. The isometric holds from previous exercise hold the movement from the up-phase of movement, the eccentric holds is holding the movement on the down phase. Hold for 5-10 seconds, relax and repeat. Remember to use the opposite arm to hold movement and keep contraction.

★★★★ Chair Curls

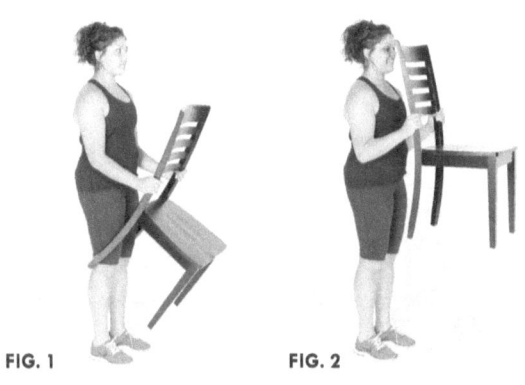

FIG. 1　　　FIG. 2

In a standing position, feet hip width apart and keep core engaged. Grab chair from a secured position, keep arms relaxed at sides, keep posture, lift chair by bending at the elbows. Lift chair from elbows, keep exercise controlled and slow contraction.

★★★★★ Assisted Bicep Curls

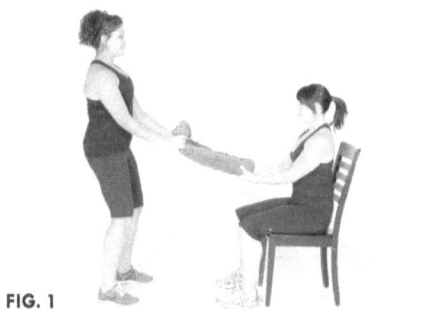

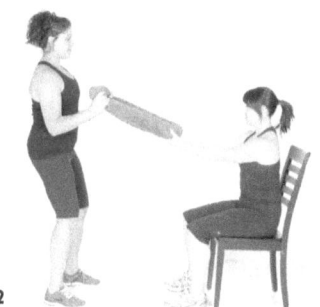

FIG. 1　　　FIG. 2

With partner and use of a towel, grip ends of towel and partner hold in the middle. The partner will give resistance as the exercisers completes exercise. Keep core activated and posture steady.

RESISTANCE TRAINING
TRICEP

Tricep movements are similar to the biceps, as in posture and contraction of the appropriate muscles need to be engaged in order to complete movement and contract the triceps. It is very important to keep shoulders back and chest up. The reason for this is because if the shoulders begin to roll forward during the exercise the body will cheat again and use the frontal shoulder and chest muscles to complete the exercise. Remember to also keep the elbows close to the body and limit it from winging out to the sides; this again will activate stronger muscles to complete the exercise. And with every exercise, remember to breathe.

MUSCLES WORKED: TRICEPS, BACK AND CORE

★ Isometric

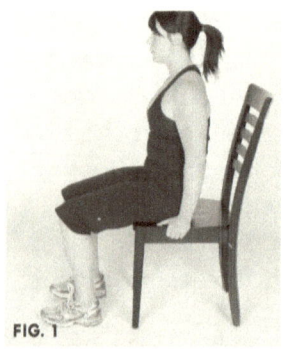 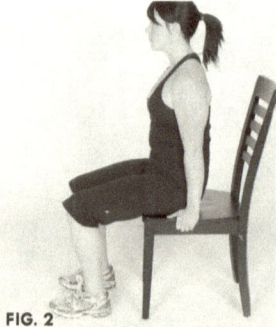

FIG. 1   FIG. 2

Seated at the edge of the chair, place hands in a comfortable position on the seat of the chair. Move weight into hands and hold 5-10 seconds, relax and repeat.

★★ Bum Dips

Seated at the edge of the chair, place hands in a comfortable position. Lift bum off seat and slowly return to starting position.

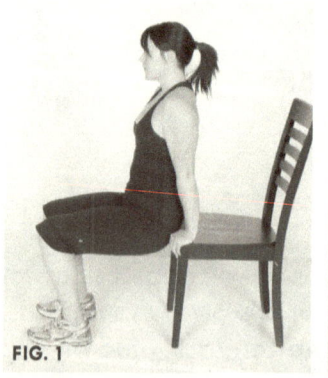 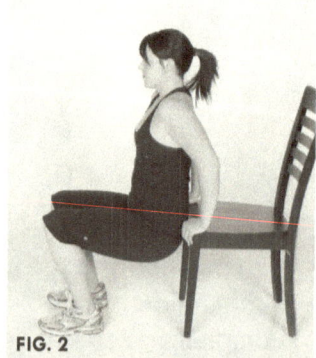

FIG. 1   FIG. 2

43

★★★ Dips Knees Bent

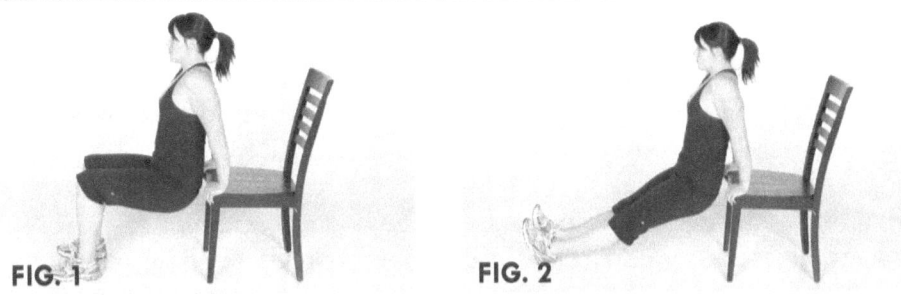

FIG. 1   FIG. 2

Sit at the edge of a chair and grip the seat of the chair with a preferred hand grip. If you have wrist problems, make sure you choose a grip that will sustain throughout the entire exercise without increase pain in your joints. Either with your knees bent or straight-legged, slide off the chair and support body weight by engaging your core muscles and keeping your elbows straight above your wrists. Lower your body weight by bending at the elbows (not at the shoulders) in a comfortable range of motion while keeping appropriate technique to sustain movement. Your elbows should stay aligned with your shoulder and not wing out. Repeat.

★★★★ Straight Legs

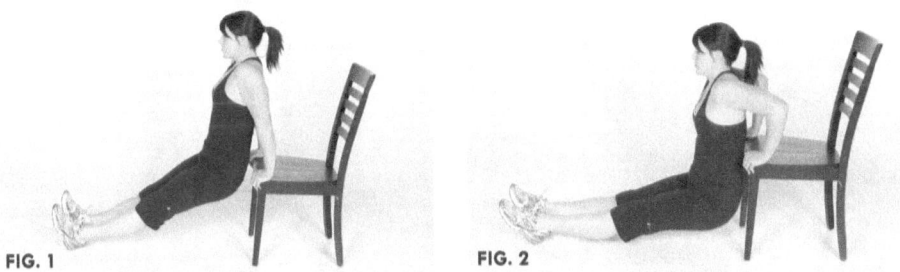

FIG. 1   FIG. 2

Same starting position as all dips, but keep legs straight, feet flexed and weight balanced on heels. Steady hand placement on chair, slide bum off seat of chair, bend elbows and lower bum in a controlled and slow business, go back to starting position and repeat.

★★★★★ One Leg

Same as straight leg dips, but with one leg, keep leg straight, and lifted. The importance is to

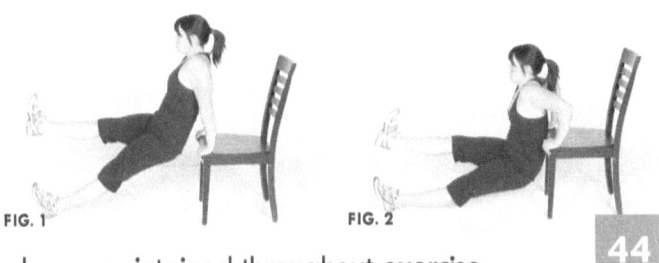

FIG. 1   FIG. 2

keep hips and core maintained throughout exercise.

44

STRETCHES

Stretching after the exercise is important to remember to do after a workout. This is to support blood circulation to the post exercise working muscles. During activity such as resistance training and cardiovascular exercise stretching is a great tool to help keep muscles limber and flexible; because, these activities helps to release toxins in the body and stretching along with circulation help eliminate these toxins. Remember a minimum of 30 seconds holding each exercise to gain the best results.

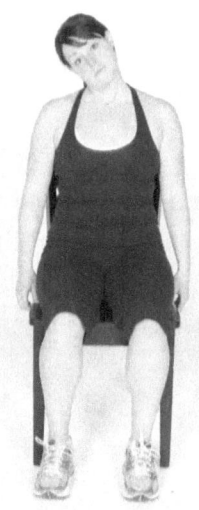

FIG. 1

FIG. 2

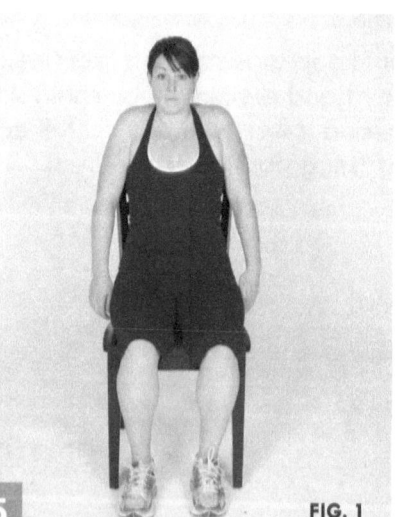

FIG. 1

FIG. 2

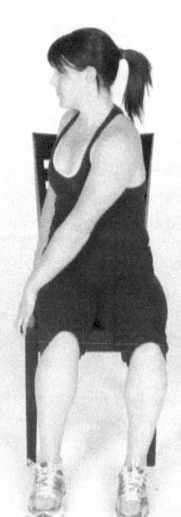

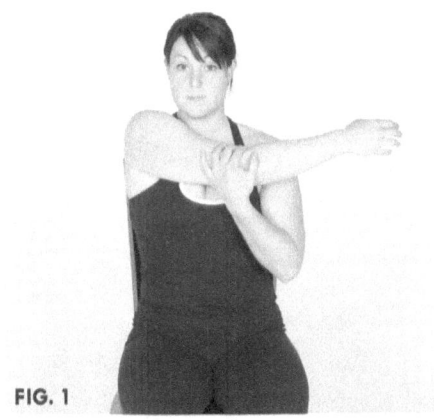

FIG. 1

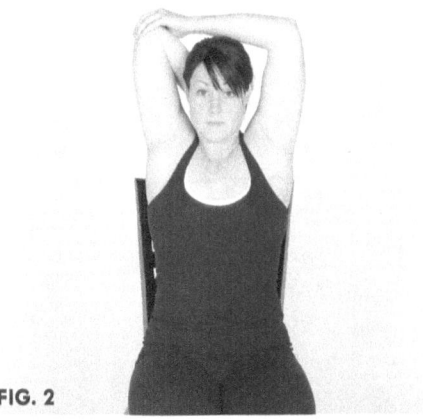

FIG. 2

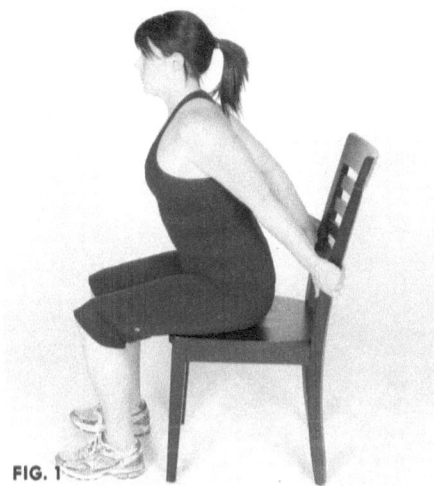

FIG. 1

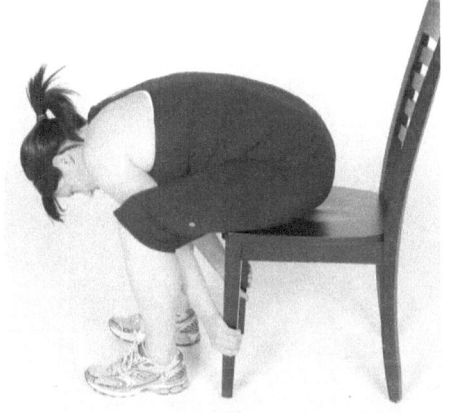

FIG. 2

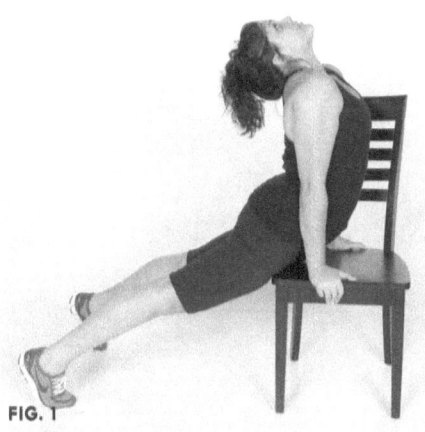

FIG. 1

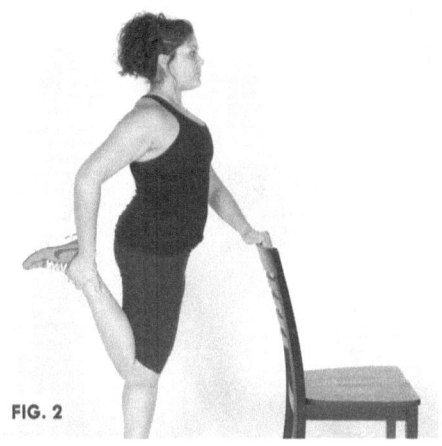

FIG. 2

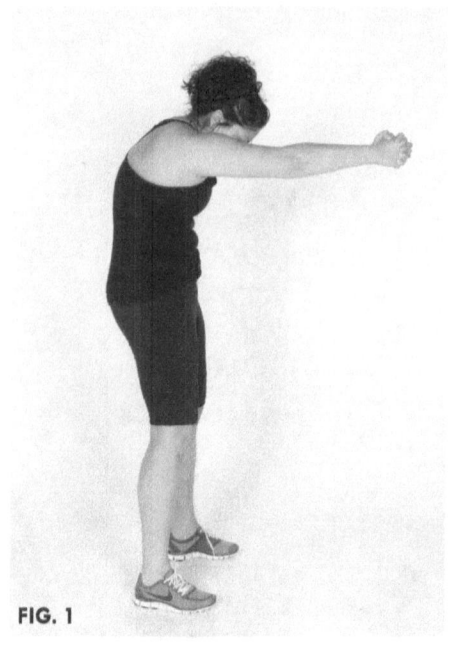

FIG. 1

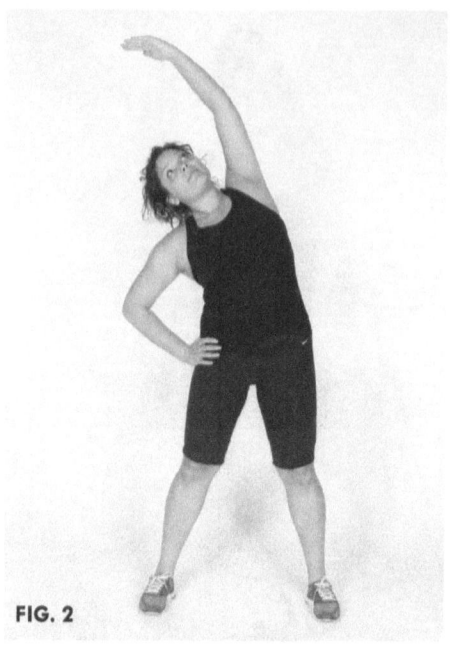

FIG. 2

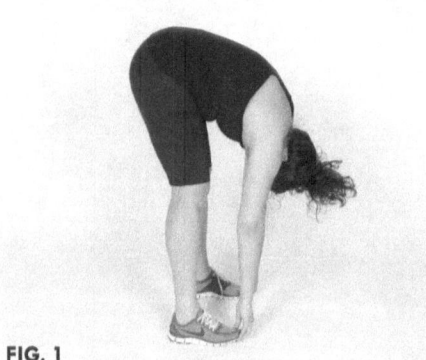

FIG. 1

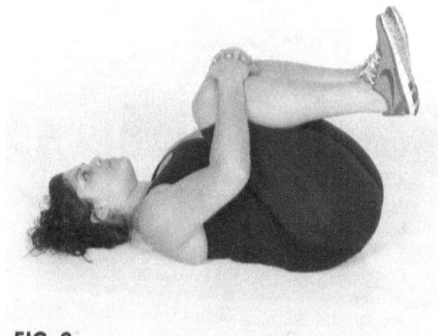

FIG. 2

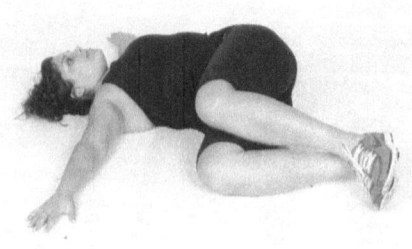

FIG. 1

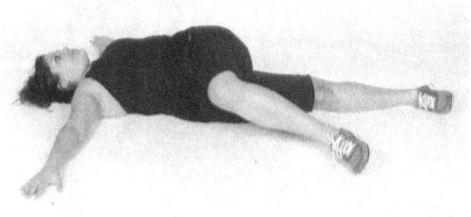

FIG. 2

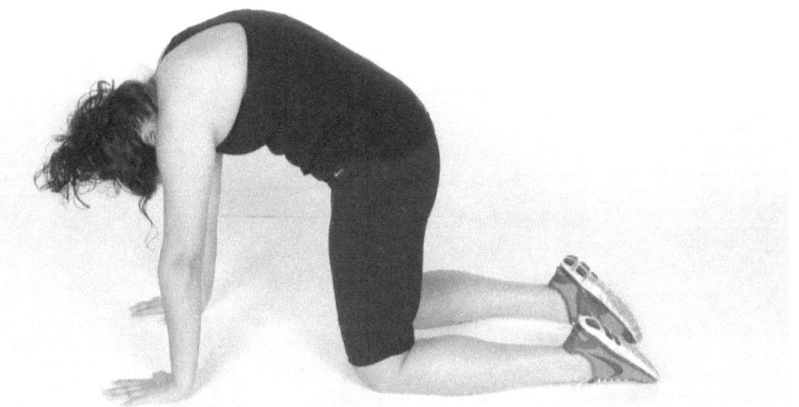

FIG. 1

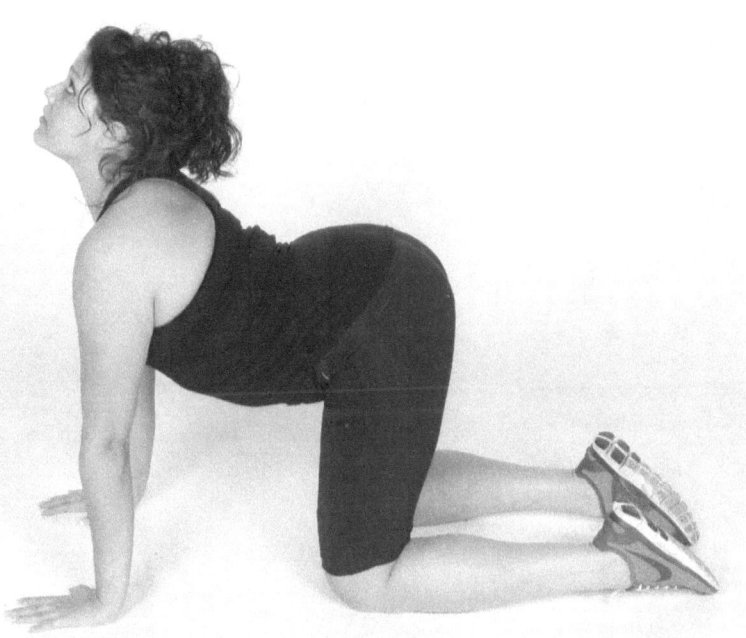

FIG. 2

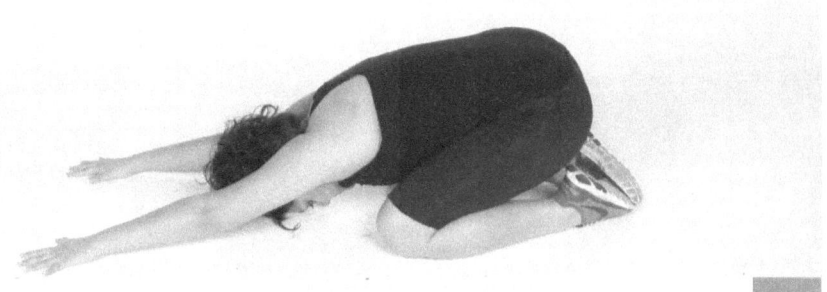

FIG. 1

Easy NUTRITION

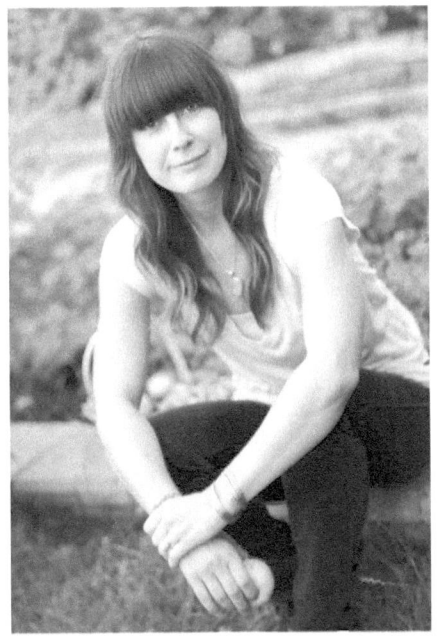

Many people think of diet as a way to trim the calories - usually for a temporary program to lose weight. What some people don't understand is that diet is not just about losing weight; it is about providing your body with the nutrition that it needs to function properly and to ward off disease and improve your inner and outer beauty. With healthy nutrition, you will feel good, look good, and improve your every day, long-term life.

Nutrition is essential to any exercise program.

Every cell in the body is being fed by the food we eat. Healthy diet is vital and it gives our body's fuel and energy to work optimally. So, it is important for us to nourish our bodies with the balance of carbohydrates, proteins, fats, vitamins, minerals and water needed for growth and repair.

There is no one diet that works for everyone, but general guidelines that can be applied to all. Eating fruits, vegetables, whole grains, legumes, proteins and healthy fats will benefit you with increased energy, weight loss, clear and strong skin, enhance moods, brain power, better sleeping habits, self esteem, staying motivated, disease prevention and overall vibrant health.

The body has extraordinary capacity to heal itself and can be done through diet alone. Refined foods, pollution, antibiotics, caffeine, stress, and a high-fat diet can impair our health and cause problems such as disease, poor immunity, digestive disorders, malabsorption of nutrients and so on.

My many years of experience working in the field of nutrition and health, I have realized that people think following a nutritional regimen is challenging and confusing. It doesn't have to be that way. EasyFit will provide you with the know-how and understanding of how easy it can be to improve your wellbeing through nutrition.

The Easy Nutrition section of this book introduces what you need to know about food and how healthy choices will benefit your everyday life.

Jennifer Hruby

ORGANIC

Why Organic?

Organic foods are higher in nutrients, free of chemicals and are grown with love. Organic foods are not grown with fertilizers, cancer-causing pesticides or growth hormones and are not processed using synthetically-produced chemicals. Foods must be evaluated and go through rigorous inspection and a set of standards in order for them to be labeled as organic. Since organic foods are free of chemicals, they taste and smell better.

LIVING FOODS (RAW)

Why Living?

Raw foods are full of enzymes that are needed to digest food to absorb the nutrients we put in our mouth. Cooking not only destroys nutrition and enzymes, but it also causes food to lose electrons—the source of energy your body needs.

ROTATION AND VARIETY

Why Rotation and Variety?

Introduce new foods weekly to fulfill your body's need for a wide range of vitamins and minerals and to avoid any deficiencies. Rotating and offering yourself a variety of foods will also ensure your diet doesn't become boring or feel like a routine.

SEASONAL FOODS

Why Seasonal?

Food that is in season is food grown right now by your local farmers. This will be fresh, better tasting food and since fewer chemicals are used, growing seasonal food is better for the environment.

NUTRITIOUS AND NATURAL

Why Nutritious and Natural?

Not packaged or frozen from the store and right from the earth will provide you with living nutrients that your body requires.

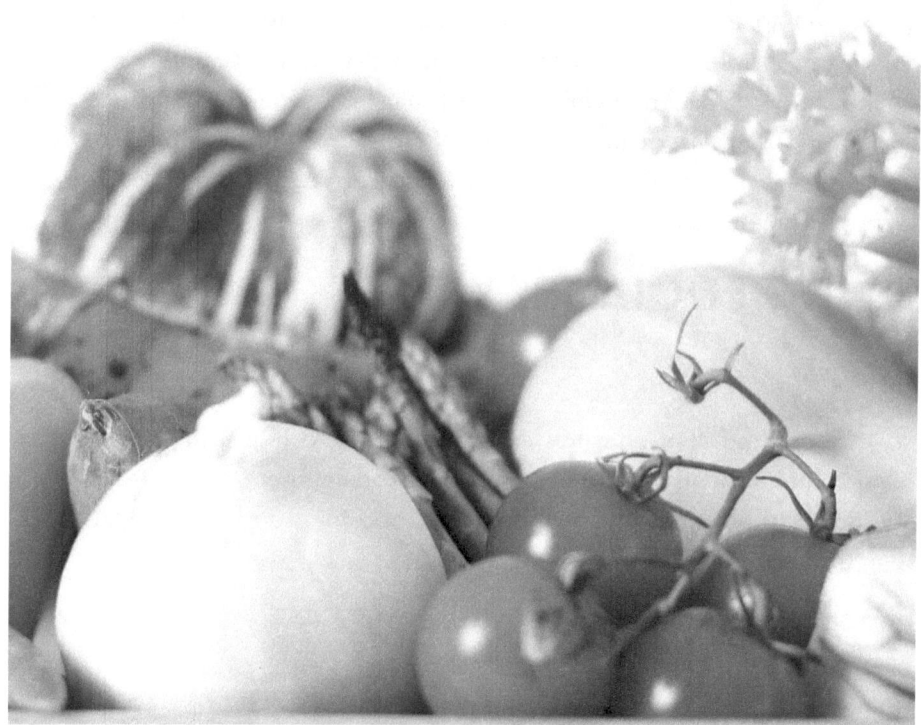

Easy Shopping and the Fundamentals

First step to shopping is deciding where to go. Start by browsing your local farmers market, the second choice would be your local health food store or grocery store. This is where you will find a bountiful amount of fresh produce. When picking out your groceries, create a rainbow in your basket loaded with colorful fresh fruits and vegetables. This prism of colour represents the variety of vitamins and minerals you will fuel your body with.

Remember, organic, raw and local. With these thoughts in mind you are supporting a greener earth, voting for better quality of life, standing by your community and decreasing your risk of disease.

53

Try new foods! Grab something you've never tried before and don't be afraid to ask people at the market or health food store how to cook or eat it. Use the Internet and search for a recipe with your chosen food. Check out YouTube on how to cook specific foods for your own personalized cooking class. There is an incredible website called 101 cookbooks that allows you to search for a recipe by ingredients. The more variety you have in your diet the less deficient you will become and the healthier you will be.

Make it an adventure or weekend activity with your family and friends. Shop together, try foods together, enjoy the atmosphere, ride your bike and then go for a picnic after with the delicious food you just picked.

When buying protein, consider visiting your local butcher for a cheaper buy. This will also provide you with a selection of meat. Try to choose lean meats like chicken, turkey and bison. With one big purchase, you can stock up your freezer to make cooking with healthy meat more convenient. When purchasing meat at the grocery store, go for organics or grain fed. Fish should be wild and not farmed. Also, when choosing your protein, remember that protein isn't only an animal source. You can buy easily digested complete protein such as quinoa, soy beans, tofu, and grains combined with nuts, seeds or beans, which have less fat than animal protein. You can also purchase powdered protein like whey or plant-based powders like rice, hemp or soy. These make for a quick shake after a workout or when in a hurry. 50 grams of complete protein a day is recommended, which is the equivalent to just over 3 tablespoons of complete protein. Yup, that is all that is required. So think twice when eating that massive steak for dinner and remember less is more.

Carbohydrates are fruit, vegetables and whole grains. 60% of your diet should be carbohydrates. They are essential and can provide remarkable energy and liveliness to one's life. Carbohydrates also strengthen your immune system, prevent irritability and help you to avoid constipation. Community gardens are a great way to get involved. By eating fresh, organic vegetables you helped grow, you gain a great appreciation for food, earth and your health. The bulk section is where you can consider buying your grains, flours, granola, nuts, seeds, and beans for a bargain price. I suggest you buy your nuts and seeds raw, which mean they have been baked, roasted, salted and are packed with nutrients. Buy a different nut every week; start with pecan, then walnut, brazil, almond, hazelnut, cashew, pine and pistachio. Try different seeds like sunflower, pumpkin, chia, flax and sesame. Add these to salads and granola, grind them and add to shakes or simply have them as a snack. When buying grains, look for spelt, amaranth, buckwheat, miller, quinoa, rice, rye and oat.

Don't forget to purchase your healthy fats. When choosing your healthy fats, remember Feed And Think Skinny! With the right kinds of fats you can effortlessly lose weight. With fats such as olive, fish, coconut, hemp, flax, oils, avocados, nuts and seeds, you are helping your body metabolize fat. You are increasing your heat production, which increases your energy that burns more calories and increases your metabolism. These fats are also known to lubricate joints, moisturize skin and speed recovery of injuries. 10 – 15 % of your diet should be fats.

When shopping for vitamins and minerals ask questions! Department store staff are educated and passionate about this subject and love to help. Like most doctors, I would suggest a multi-vitamin or even a "greens" supplement. Antioxidants are essential for fighting free-radical damage caused by toxins and are crucial for anti-aging and longevity. Essential fatty acids are not made by the body and need to be supplemented.

*any gas or bloating - enzymes or probiotics
*fiber supplement

Easy Eating

Think of food as a source of income. The abundance of nutritious food you feed your body, the richer you are in health. Believe it or not, it can be easy so start investing!

Start with visualization. Visualize your abundance and what it will bring to your life - looking youthful, having energy to do more every day, setting an example, fitting back into those old jeans you loved so much and having the metabolism you had many years ago. Visualize that these desires are possible.

The importance of easy eating is staying positive and focused.

Focus on what you CAN eat rather than what you cannot. Imagine delicious, nutritious, colorful, organic foods that will benefit you and your future.

Steps to easy eating are as follows:

- Menu planning
- Preparation
- Creativeness, and
- Learning

Menu Planning

Menu planning will eliminate those stressful headaches of decision making and last-minute binge eating. Take an hour out of your week and carefully plan a week or two of an array of nutritious meals. This can also be done daily. A few minutes before you go to bed or first thing in the morning, plan your meals for the day. That simple.

Along with your menu plan, we are going to incorporate your goals. A good way to see results is to start with a calendar and a package of stickers. Any stickers will do and you can find a variety at your local dollar store. On the days you follow your menu plan, give yourself a sticker for achievement. This will give you a clear picture of your eating patterns and if your goals are being reached. It will also help motivate you for success. Keep in mind your positive outlook. If your week is looking a little bare with no stickers, hang in there and make next week a 7-star week. Later in this book, we will go through examples of what a menu plan should look like.

Preparation

Preparing meals ahead of time is important and helps you avoid leaving your home without a packed lunch and snacks. After your trip to the grocery store, you should prepare meals for the week. Clean your fridge out and start chopping. Pre-cook or sprout your grains, wash and cut all your vegetables and place them in containers.

Plan your cravings! Sometimes they are unavoidable, so prepare healthy and guilt-free choices for when that time comes. You can store dark chocolate or rice, coconut and soy ice cream in the freezer. An alternative to a healthy ice cream is pre-making smoothie popsicles. Pre-bake healthy deserts with ingredients like tahini, maple syrup, agave nectar, oats, nuts, applesauce, dried fruits and grains.

Creativeness

Be creative and have fun with your food. Introduce this way of living to your friends, family and employees. Plan potluck lunches, exchange recipes and even collect recipes and create a personalized cookbook. Introduce it to your community and share ideas, literature and healthy tips. Get yourself an apron and have fun.

Learning

Learning about nutrition makes life easier. Living a healthy life and staying out of the doctor's office is your responsibility, so get involved. Get some books, surf the net and ask questions. Visit your local farms and learn how they grow their food or raise their animals. Pick a vegetable or fruit of the week and look up the vitamins and minerals it serves. Pick a grain you've never cooked or baked with. Sprout! This is a fascinating experience and a great way to incorporate enzymes that are needed for digestion and absorption. Call up a Holistic Nutritionist and plan a workshop or a cooking class. The more educated you are about nutrition, the more you understand what you should and shouldn't eat and why. Get inspired and enjoy the benefits.

Sample Menu Plan

Breakfast

Breakfast is the most important meal of your day. For time-released energy, start your day
with the following:

- granola with nuts, seeds, dried fruit, hemp hearts and chia seeds
- whole-grain cereal with Almond or Rice milk
    - warm oatmeal with cinnamon, honey and flax

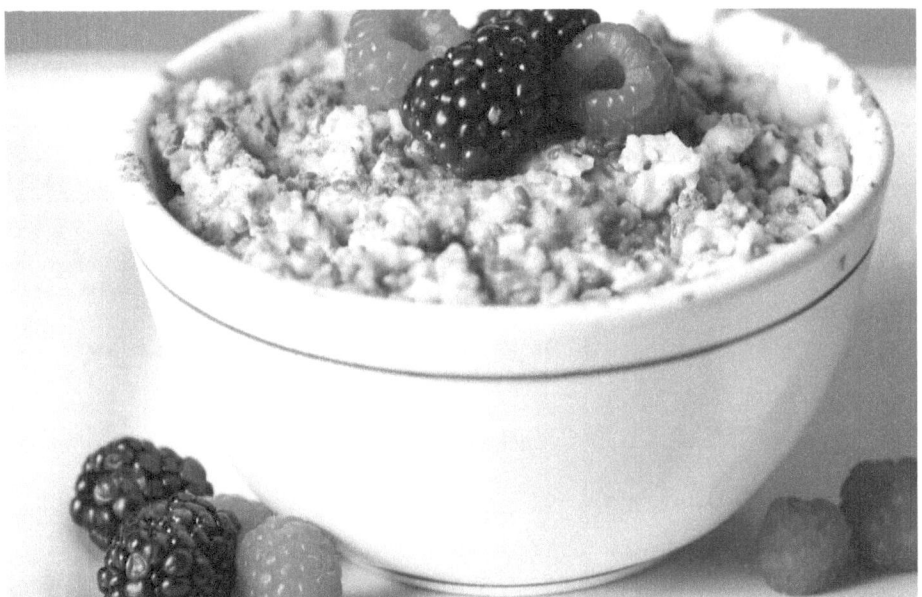

Snacks

Snacks are important to keep your blood sugar balanced, and provide energy which also aids in weight loss.

- trail mix
- protein smoothie
- hard boiled eggs and cucumbers

Lunch

Lunch is a good time to eat your protein. Animal protein takes a long time to digest and that is why it is better eaten at lunch rather than dinner. It is also a good time to fuel up.

- chicken with steamed vegetables drizzled with some olive oil and sesame seeds
- salmon and a salad with a copious amount of vegetables
- quinoa salad with carrots, pumpkin seeds, hemp oil and cayenne pepper
- brown rice with beans and garlicky zucchini

Snack

A light snack is great for an energy boost.

EASY BREEZY SHOPPING LIST

Vegetables		Grains	Raw nuts and seeds	
Red, green, yellow, orange peppers	Potato	Spelt	Cashews	Walnuts
	Radish	Rye		
Carrots	Bok Choy		Almonds	Pumpkin
Eggplant	Asparagus	Millet		
Turnips	Artichoke		Brazil nuts	Sunflower
Squash	Onions	Quinoa		
Pumpkin	Tomato	Buckwheat	Hazelnuts	Chia
Broccoli	Cabbage			
Cauliflower	Brussel Sprouts	Oats	Pecans	Flax
Beets		Kamut		
Beans	Kale		Pistachios	Sesame
Green Peas	Spinach	Barley		
Okra	Swiss Chard			
Yam	Collards	Amaranth		
Zucchini	Watercress	Brown Rice		

Beans	Fruit	
Soybeans	Apples	Dragon Fruit
	Bananas	Mangosteen
Aduki	Kiwi	Apricots
	Mango	Cherries
Mung	Cranberries	Grapes
	Dates	Guavas
Black beans	Grapefruit	Lychees
	Oranges	Nectarines
Garbanzo	Lemons	Peaches
	Limes	Papaya
Lentils	Pineapples	Pears
Navy	Strawberries	Cantaloupe
	Blueberries	Honeydew
Lima	Pomegranates	Watermelon
Fava	Passion Fruit	Raspberries

- carrots and cucumbers
- rice cakes and almond butter
- rice crackers and toffuti (tofu cream cheese, delicious!)

Dinner

A light, nutritious dinner is easy to digest before bedtime.
Note: For a restful sleep, meals should be eaten 3-4 hours before bedtime.

- spelt pasta with a blend of vegetables, plus olive oil, salt and pepper, and fresh herbs

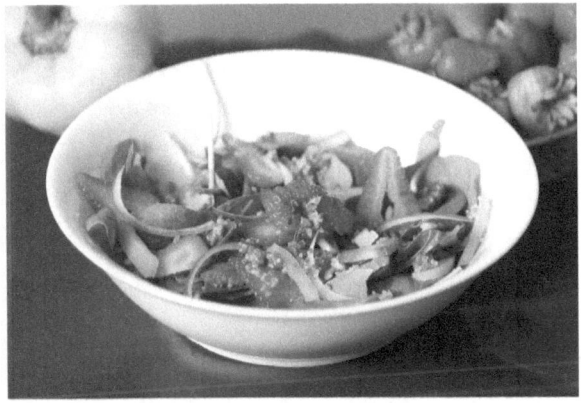

- vegetarian chili with beans and barley

- baked root vegetables with beans and brown rice

- vegetarian bean wraps with spinach and homemade salsa

The Spunk on Detox

When I think of detoxing, I relate my body to a vacuum. When a vacuum stops running smoothly it means the filter needs to be emptied. When our energy level starts to slow down this is a sign our body functions also need a little clean up and expulsion. The buildup of toxins from pollution, cigarette smoke, food additives, alcohol, carbonated sodas, white sugar and processed food can be damaging to our body. Detoxing is simple and can be done on a daily basis.

When you rise in the morning, start your day off with a glass of water with lemon. This will get your mucus moving and kick-start your digestive juices. Before eating breakfast, consume a piece of fruit. Cleansing fruits are apples, apricots, lemons, peaches and berries. These fruits are full of antioxidants and fuel our metabolism. Fruit like apples are high in fiber and low in calories. Fiber binds to toxins and heavy metals that help cleanse the colon. Legumes are also loaded with fiber, low in fat, a good protein source, and needed to balance sugar levels and lower cholesterol. Legumes are peas, beans and lentils--add them to brown rice and you have yourself a complete protein. This is very important for vegetarians to understand since some vegetarians may not be getting enough protein in their diet. Drink heaps of water throughout the day. Water is needed for our bodily functions to work properly. Drink herbal teas like dandelion, nettle, licorice, ginger and fennel—these herbs are a natural diuretic, they help with digestion, work as an anti-inflammatory and a mild laxative. Try a green drink! Blend green veggies with an apple or orange to sweeten it up. Juicing greens delivers an ample amount of vitamins, nutrients and cleansing properties.

Get Your Skinny on With These Tips and Tricks

Now it's time to relax, stop counting calories and encourage awareness. We need to adjust your taste buds, manifest your goals and take action. Here are some tips on increasing your metabolism and weight loss:

- Cayenne   this spice speeds up metabolism and balances sugar levels. It aids in elimination and helps in healing the stomach

- Flax oil   attracts oil soluble toxins and removes them from the body, a calorie burner and is also good for immune and cardiovascular help

- Probiotics   healthy bacteria that keeps the intestinal track working at its best for better digestion, absorption and elimination, also helps immunity and disease prevention

- Cinnamon   is the spice we think could be bad but is very beneficial in metabolizing sugar, excess sugar contributes to weight gain

- Green Vegetables   a good source of fiber and packed with beneficial vitamins and antioxidants that your body craves, and when you give your body what it needs, it helps prevent cravings of the bad food and helps prevent hunger

- Garlic and onions   these two miracle workers have phytochemicals that break down fatty deposits, these are super foods for immunity and garllic acts as a natural antibiotic

- Olive oil   can curb cravings and when getting this right kind of fat your body is satisfied. Cravings occur when your body requires something that is missing in the diet. That is why it is important to have a balanced diet that includes fats. Olive oil is also really good for your skin and hair.

- Beans   a good source of fiber, which stabilizes blood sugar levels, prevents cravings and helps aid in weight loss

Easy Weight Loss

Let's make weight loss meaningful! Think of the abundance of healthy food that surround you and focus on positive influence. Instantly introduce "healthy thought" to your life and commit to incorporating it into your daily diet. Attract strength and manifest your goals.

Cherish your life, accept change and make it easy.

Easy weight loss starts with monitoring what you eat, when you eat it and how you feel. So grab a notebook, decorate it with love and start writing! Add quotes, affirmations, pictures and drawings—anything that will inspire you and your journey to change.

Easy Weight Loss Tips

1. Start by eating smaller meals every couple hours. This will increase your metabolism and balance your blood sugar. When your blood sugar is balanced your cravings diminish, your energy increases and you boost your brain activity.
2. Start your day with a breakfast full of nuts, seeds, oats, and flax for slow-released energy. It's a great way to jump-start your day.
3. Snack on foods that are nutritious and feed your body energy.
4. Snack on protein foods to balance sugar levels and help with weight loss. Hard-boiled eggs, nuts and seeds, almond butter, cottage cheese, quinoa are great sources of protein.
   5. Alkalize your body! This will increase energy, assist in weight loss and prevent disease.

6. Add enzymes to your diet. For proper digestion, absorption and elimination, you need to digest your food properly. This will increase your metabolism and energy.
7. Add raw foods and sprouted seeds to your regimen. These foods are full of nutrients and enzymes.
8. Do not drink fluids with your meals. If you drink fluids while eating, your body's digestive enzymes won't perform their job in helping with digestion.
9. Help digestion with supplementing enzymes.
10. Yerba mate – suppresses hunger, increases metabolism
11. Try gluten-free foods. A lot of people have sensitivity to it.
12. Try not eating red meat.
13. Apple cider vinegar – good for digestion, reduce bloating
14. Food combining
15. Eat slowly. The more you chew your food the better it digests and more is absorbed causing you to get fuller faster. Overeating can cause stress to the digestion system.
16. Alcohol weakens the metabolism and increases bad eating.
17. EFAs plus protein help curb cravings

Easy Water Drinking

Hydrate your cells! Water is needed for all bodily fluids and functions, circulation, digestion, absorption, and elimination. Toxins need to be flushed through urine and sweat, so in order for this process to work, you need to drink water. Required amount is said to be around.

Easy Snacks
- popcorn with coconut butter
- yogurt with added milled flax seeds, nuts and berries
- apple with a nut butter
- turkey or salmon jerky
- poached egg with veggies
- sprouts
- trail mix - add dried apricots or cranberries, nuts, seeds and carob junks
- hummus or guacamole and veggies
    - baked chickpeas
    - kale chips

Easy Recipes for Easy Eating

EASY BELOVED MANGO INSPIRATION
- 1 part millet
- 2 parts water
- raw sunflower Seeds
- raw pecans
- milled flax
- mango

Boil 1 part millet to 2 parts water and simmer until water is absorbed into the millet. Place in a bowl and add raw sunflower seeds, raw pecans, milled flax and mango.

Autumn flavored squash
- 1 acorn squash
- olive oil
- thyme
- rosemary
- lentils or brown rice

Set the oven to 350 degrees. Cut an acorn squash into cube pieces. Cover baking sheet with olive oil and sprinkle thyme and rosemary. Place the acorn on a sheet and bake for about 45 minutes or until squash is soft and a little browned. Add to lentils that have been steamed in a rice cooker or brown rice.

INDULGING MEATLESS TACO
- 1 can of black beans
- 2 cups of brown rice
- 1 red or yellow pepper
- 1 tomato
- 1 red or yellow onion
- salt and pepper to taste
- cayenne
- cumin
- olive oil
- garlic
- spinach
- avocado
- yogurt
- old-aged cheese
- taco shells

Add beans, peppers, tomato, onion, garlic, spices, olive oil and blend in a food processor or magic bullet. Put mashed ingredients on the bottom of a taco shell, then top with rice, spinach, avocado and cheese.

* Cayenne is good for boosting metabolism.
* Brown rice is high in B vitamins and selenium, which is essential for healthy skin, hair and nails and also protects against free radicals.
* Avocados are rich in Vitamin A, C and E.
* Garlic is a natural antibiotic and helps ward off infections, fungus and helps with immunity, digestion and circulation.

BEET SOUPALICIOUS

This recipe is a great fall and winter soup.

- 3 beets
- 2 carrots
- 1 medium onion
- 2 garlic cloves
- 2 tablespoons of olive oil
- 1 yam
- 1 turnip
- bouillon of choice
- dill (optional)
- salt and pepper to taste
- cayenne

Sauté the onion with olive oil until browned. Add garlic and sauté for another minute. Add chopped carrots, yam and turnip. Sauté for about 3 more minutes and then add enough water to fill a big soup pot (about 2 inches from the brim). Add bouillon and bring to a boil. Simmer and cook until you can put a fork through the carrots. In a food processor, blend all vegetables and put back into the pot. Put beets in the food processer and mix until pureed and add to soup. Cook for another 5 minutes. Add cayenne, salt and pepper. Pour into bowl and garnish with fresh dill.

Easy Eating Out

Tips when eating out

- Don't drink fluids with your dinner.
- Stay away from fried foods.
- Get your dressing on the side and try a healthy vinaigrette.

- Order a healthy salad as a appetizer, side or as your meal
- Customize your meal! Ask the server to not add sauce or salt.
- Skip the dessert or order fruit instead.
- Don't order saucy meals like Fettuccine Alfredo or stir fry's.

Easy Energy

During my past experience working at health food stores, the biggest complaint I got was people experiencing lack of energy.

Greens, algae, grains, sprouts, vegetables, wheat grass, essential fatty acids (lubricate your colon), B-vitamins, poor adrenals, metabolism-boosting nutrients - vitamin C, magnesium, zinc, iron, co 10 and the herbal plant astragalus. vitamin C

Recipes and Food Ideas

- granola pie
- zuchini hummus
- pumpkin hummus
- cauliflower hummus
- bison sheppard pie
- veg tacos
- raw energy bars
- homemade ketchup
- sweet potatoe salad
- summer red cabbage salad
- millet breakie

Bad Foods - Danger

- Sugar is an addiction and causes illness, mood swings, irritability, weight gain, depression, anxiety and tooth decay. Sugar and highly processed foods can actually wipe out vitamins and minerals from the body. Sugar is atrocious to our immunity and causes imbalance.

- Toxins overwork the liver. When the liver has too much toxins to handle, they get deposited into your tissues.
  Ensure you take flax oil.

- Caffeine causes anxiety, makes the body very acidic, which causes disease and also stresses the immune system. Try yerba mate or green tea which aid in weight loss.

- Overeating causes great stress on the body and sedates organs. It reduces nutrient absorption and the body craves more food because it is malnourished.

- Examples of bad carbohydrates that you should not eat are cakes, cookies and sweets.

www.ingramcontent.com/pod-product-compliance
Lightning Source LLC
Chambersburg PA
CBHW021247280526
45784CB00005B/2275